Updates in Geriatric Nephrology

Editors

EDGAR V. LERMA
MITCHELL H. ROSNER

CLINICS IN
GERIATRIC MEDICINE

www.geriatric.theclinics.com

August 2013 • Volume 29 • Number 3

ELSEVIER

1600 John F. Kennedy Boulevard • Suite 1800 • Philadelphia, Pennsylvania, 19103-2899

http://www.theclinics.com

CLINICS IN GERIATRIC MEDICINE Volume 29, Number 3
August 2013 ISSN 0749–0690, ISBN-13: 978-0-323-18604-9

Editor: Yonah Korngold

Clinics in Geriatric Medicine (ISSN 0749-0690) is published quarterly by Elsevier Inc., 360 Park Avenue South, New York, NY 10010-1710. Months of issue are February, May, August, and November. Business and Editorial Offices: 1600 John F. Kennedy Blvd., Suite 1800, Philadelphia, PA 191023-2899. Periodicals postage paid at New York, NY, and additional mailing offices. Subscription prices are $269.00 per year (US individuals), $475.00 per year (US institutions), $137.00 per year (US student/resident), $350.00 per year (Canadian individuals), $591.00 per year (Canadian institutions), $186.00 per year (Canadian student/resident), $372.00 per year (foreign individuals), $591.00 per year (foreign institutions), and $186.00 per year (foreign student/resident). Foreign air speed delivery is included in all *Clinics* subscription prices. All prices are subject to change without notice. POSTMASTER: Send address changes to *Clinics in Geriatric Medicine,* Elsevier Health Sciences Division, Subscription Customer Service, 3251 Riverport Lane, Maryland Heights, MO 63043. Telephone: 1-800-654-2452 (U.S. and Canada); 314-447-8871 (outside U.S. and Canada). Fax: 314-447-8029. E-mail: journalscustomerservice-usa@elsevier.com (for print support) or journalsonlinesupport-usa@elsevier.com (for online support).

Reprints. For copies of 100 or more, of articles in this publication, please contact the Commercial Reprints Department, Elsevier Inc., 360 Park Avenue South, New York, New York 10010-1710. Tel.: (212) 633-3812; Fax: (212) 462-1935, email: reprints@elsevier.com.

Clinics in Geriatric Medicine is covered in *MEDLINE/PubMed (Index Medicus), EMBASE/Excerpta Medica, Current Contents/Clinical Medicine (CC/CM),* and the *Cumulative Index to Nursing & Allied Health Literature.*

Printed and bound by CPI Group (UK) Ltd, Croydon, CR0 4YY

Transferred to digital print 2013

Contributors

EDITORS

EDGAR V. LERMA, MD, FACP, FASN, FAHA, FASH, FNLA, FNKF
Clinical Professor of Medicine, Section of Nephrology, University of Illinois at Chicago
College of Medicine, Chicago, Illinois; Educational Coordinator for Nephrology,
UIC - Advocate Christ Medical Center, Oak Lawn, Illinois

MITCHELL H. ROSNER, MD, FACP
Chairman, Department of Medicine, Henry B. Mulholland Professor of Medicine, Division
of Nephrology, University of Virginia Health System, Charlottesville, Virgninia

AUTHORS

EMAAD M. ABDEL-RAHMAN, MD, PhD
Professor, Division of Nephrology, University of Virginia, Charlottesville, Virginia

RASHEED A. BALOGUN, MD
Associate Professor, Division of Nephrology, University of Virginia, Charlottesville, Virginia

WILLIAM M. BENNETT, MD
Clinical Transplant, Northwest Renal Clinic, Legacy Good Samaritan Hospital Transplant
Services, Portland, Oregon

MARKUS BITZER, MD
Assistant Professor, Division of Nephrology, Internal Medicine, University of Michigan,
Ann Arbor, Michigan

LINDA FRIED, MD, MPH
Staff Physician, Renal Section, VA Pittsburgh Healthcare System; Professor of Medicine,
Epidemiology, and Clinical and Translational Science, University of Pittsburgh, Pittsburgh,
Pennsylvania

RICHARD J. GLASSOCK, MD
Emeritus Professor, Department of Medicine, The David Geffen School of Medicine,
UCLA, Laguna Niguel, Los Angeles, California

SARBJIT VANITA JASSAL, MB, MD, FRCPC
Associate Professor of Medicine, Division of Nephrology, Department of Medicine,
University of Toronto, University Health Network, Toronto, Ontario, Canada

ZEINA KARAM, MD
Fellow, Division of Nephrology and Hypertension, Northwestern University Feinberg
School of Medicine, Chicago, Illinois

DOUGLAS SCOTT KEITH, MD
Associate Professor of Medicine, Division of Nephrology, Department of Medicine,
University of Virginia Medical Center, Charlottesville, Virginia

HOLLY M. KONCICKI, MD, MS
Fellow, Nephrology, Department of Medicine; Department of Geriatrics and Palliative Medicine, Icahn School of Medicine at Mount Sinai, New York, New York

JESSICA LASSITER, PharmD, BCPS
Department of Pharmacy Services, University of Michigan Hospital and Health Systems, Ann Arbor, Michigan

TUSCHAR MALAVADE, MD, DNB
Clinical Fellow, Division of Nephrology, Department of Medicine, University of Toronto, University Health Network, Toronto, Ontario, Canada

THIN THIN MAW, MBBS, MS
Nephrology Fellow, Renal-Electrolyte Division, University of Pittsburgh School of Medicine, Pittsburgh, Pennsylvania

ALI J. OLYAEI, PharmD
Professor of Medicine, Division of Nephrology & Hypertension, Oregon State University and Oregon Health & Sciences University, Portland, Oregon

MITCHELL H. ROSNER, MD, FACP
Chairman, Department of Medicine, Henry B. Mulholland Professor of Medicine, Division of Nephrology, University of Virginia Health System, Charlottesville, Virgninia

AHMED SOKWALA, MD
Clinical Fellow, Division of Nephrology, Department of Medicine, University of Toronto, University Health Network, Toronto, Ontario, Canada

MARK A. SWIDLER, MD
Associate Professor, Nephrology, Department of Medicine; Department of Geriatrics and Palliative Medicine, Icahn School of Medicine at Mount Sinai, New York, New York

JENNIFER TUAZON, MD
Assistant Professor, Division of Nephrology and Hypertension, Northwestern University Feinberg School of Medicine, Chicago, Illinois

FARUK TURGUT, MD
Associate Professor, Department of Nephrology, School of Medicine, Mustafa Kemal University, Hatay, Turkey

JOCELYN WIGGINS, B.M., B.Ch, MRCP
Associate Professor, Division of Geriatrics, Internal Medicine, University of Michigan, Ann Arbor, Michigan

YUSUF YESIL, MD
Division of Geriatric Medicine, Department of Internal Medicine, School of Medicine, Hacettepe University, Ankara, Turkey

Contents

Aging is associated with structural and functional changes in the kidney. Structural changes include glomerulosclerosis, thickening of the basement membrane, increase in mesangial matrix, tubulointerstitial fibrosis and arteriosclerosis. Glomerular filtration rate is maintained until the fourth decade of life, after which it declines. Parallel reductions in renal blood flow occur with redistribution of blood flow from the cortex to the medulla. Other functional changes include an increase in glomerular basement permeability and decreased ability to dilute or concentrate urine.

Most patients who develop acute kidney injury (AKI) are older than 65 years. Specific structural and functional changes that occur in the aging kidney predispose the elderly patient to AKI. This risk is further compounded by comorbid conditions, polypharmacy, and the need for invasive procedures. When AKI does occur, it is associated with significant morbidity and mortality. Although morbidity and mortality increases with advancing age, many elderly patients can survive AKI and do well. Thus, decision making should be thoughtful and individualized, and not dependent on age. Whenever possible, preventive approaches should be pursued to lessen the burden of AKI.

Examination of urinary sediment for dysmorphic erythrocytes as a diagnostic tool in glomerular disease is important. The atypical clinical features of acute and chronic glomerular disease in the elderly should be remembered. The common causes of nephrotic syndrome need to be remembered in patients with edema and marked proteinuria. The predilection of the elderly to develop rapidly progressive glomerulonephritis needs to be appreciated. The development of glomerular disease caused by an underlying neoplastic process also needs to be remembered. Effective treatment regimens are available to ameliorate the adverse consequences of acute, progressive, and chronic glomerular disease in the geriatric population.

Elderly individuals, worldwide, are on the rise, posing new challenges to care providers. Hypertension is highly prevalent in elderly individuals, and multiple challenges face care providers while managing it. In addition to treating hypertension, the physician must treat other modifiable cardiovascular risk factors in patients with or without diabetes mellitus or chronic kidney disease to reduce cardiovascular events and mortality. This review discusses some of the unique characteristics of high blood pressure in the elderly and provides an overview of the challenges facing care providers, as well as the current recommendations for management of hypertension in the elderly.

Chronic kidney disease (CKD) is increasingly being recognized as a disease of elderly individuals. In recent years the definition and categorization of kidney disease has been standardized. There are concerns that this standardization has led to an increase in the number of older individuals labeled as having CKD. This article addresses the definitions of CKD, recently published revised CKD stages with risk stratifications, and limitations of using formulas to assess renal function in the elderly. Also discussed are management of common risk factors of progression CKD, nonrenal-related outcomes, prognosis of CKD in older individuals, and criteria for referral to nephrology.

Each year a large number of older individuals with advanced renal disease are started on chronic dialysis therapy. Life expectancy is estimated at between 2 and 4 years depending on age, comorbidity, and intensity of medical care required in the weeks around the dialysis start time. Survivors remain at high risk of ongoing morbidity. Regarding quality of life, many older patients express regret over having opted for chronic dialysis therapy and subsequently choose to withdraw from treatment, whereas many others maintain a quality of life similar to that of age-matched peers. Early assessment and ongoing comprehensive geriatric assessment is recommended.

Because the fastest-growing group of patients undergoing dialysis is older than 75 years, geriatricians will be more involved in decisions regarding the appropriate treatment of end-stage renal disease. A thoughtful approach to shared decision making regarding dialysis or nondialysis medical therapy (NDMT) includes consideration of medical indications, patient preferences, quality of life, and contextual features. Determination of prognosis and expected performance on dialysis based on disease trajectories and assessment of functional age should be shared with patients and families. The Renal Physician Association's guidelines on shared decision making in dialysis offer recommendations to help with dialysis or NDMT decisions.

CLINICS IN GERIATRIC MEDICINE

Preface

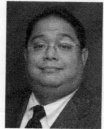
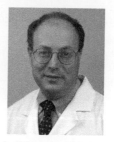

Edgar V. Lerma, MD, FACP, FASN, FAHA, FASH, FNLA, FNKF   Mitchell H. Rosner, MD, FACP
Editors

The changing demographics of the global population predict that the number of people age 65 years or greater will triple over the coming decades. This reflects improvements in medical care, living conditions, nutrition, and many other factors. Because the incidence and prevalence of kidney disease increase with advancing age, clinicians will be confronted with an elderly population of patients that have disease affecting the kidneys as well as other comorbid conditions at higher and higher rates. Furthermore, it is more and more understood that it requires a specific knowledge set to effectively address the unique problems that result from aging in nephrologic diagnosis and treatment.

This issue of *Clinics in Geriatric Medicine* focuses on the kidney. The issue begins with a description of the key anatomic and physiologic changes in the kidney that are associated with aging. This understanding is critical in deciphering the various syndromes of kidney disease that are manifest in the elderly population. Topics such as acute kidney injury and glomerular disease in the elderly focus on the unique aspects of these syndromes in older patients. Other key topics include unique management issues in the hypertensive elderly patient as well as chronic kidney disease and end-stage renal disease management in the geriatric patient. Drug-dosing, which is a challenge in the older patient with kidney disease, is discussed in depth. The controversial topic of kidney transplantation is covered as well as the critical issues surrounding decision-making in elderly patients with complex medical problems. Finally, there is a provocative discussion on slowing the aging process.

Clin Geriatr Med 29 (2013) ix–x
http://dx.doi.org/10.1016/j.cger.2013.06.001
0749-0690/13/$ – see front matter © 2013 Elsevier Inc. All rights reserved.

geriatric.theclinics.com

We hope that this issue will provide clinicians with the key knowledge to care for elderly patients across a spectrum of kidney disease.

Edgar V. Lerma, MD, FACP, FASN, FAHA, FASH, FNLA, FNKF
Section of Nephrology
University of Illinois at Chicago College of Medicine
1853 West Polk Street
Chicago, IL 60612, USA

UIC - Advocate Christ Medical Center
Oak Lawn, Illinois, USA

Mitchell H. Rosner, MD, FACP
Department of Medicine
University of Virginia Health System
Charlottesville, VA 22908, USA

E-mail addresses:
nephron0@gmail.com (E.V. Lerma)
MHR9R@hscmail.mcc.virginia.edu (M.H. Rosner)

Anatomic and Physiologic Changes of the Aging Kidney

Zeina Karam, MD, Jennifer Tuazon, MD*

KEYWORDS

- Senescence • Glomerulosclerosis • Glomerular filtration rate • Renal mass
- Renin-angiotensin system • Renal blood flow • Functional reserve • Osmoregulation

KEY POINTS

- Kidney mass declines with age.
- Compensation of functional nephrons preserves kidney volume.
- The number of functional glomeruli declines with normal aging.
- Glomerular size increases and glomerular density decreases with aging.
- Normal aging is accompanied by glomerulosclerosis, tubular atrophy, arteriosclerosis, and interstitial fibrosis.
- Common histologic changes include loss of afferent and efferent arterioles in the cortex and shunting of the renal blood flow to the medulla.
- Glomerular filtration rate declines with normal aging.
- There is an increase in glomerular basement membrane permeability, resulting in an increase in urinary excretion of proteins.
- Both the diluting and concentrating ability is reduced.

Aging is a complex process driven by various molecular pathways and biochemical events that result in significant changes in all organs. In the kidneys, aging is associated with structural and physiologic changes. There is a linear relationship between aging and a decline in renal function. The rate of decline varies with sex, ethnicity, and comorbidities. Renal function is estimated to decline by a mean of 0.75 mL/min per year even in the absence of comorbidities such as diabetes and hypertension.[1]

With advancing age, the kidneys undergo anatomic and physiologic changes, with a notable decline in glomerular filtration rate (GFR) and a variation in the ability to respond to acute changes and maintain kidney function. Whether the decline in creatinine clearance with aging is a physiologic process or whether it is secondary to diseases that become more prevalent with aging remains an issue of debate.

Disclosures: None.
Division of Nephrology and Hypertension, Northwestern University Feinberg School of Medicine, 710 North Fairbanks Court, Olson 4-500, Chicago, IL 60611, USA
* Corresponding author.
E-mail address: j-tuazon@northwestern.edu

Clin Geriatr Med 29 (2013) 555–564
http://dx.doi.org/10.1016/j.cger.2013.05.006
0749-0690/13/$ – see front matter © 2013 Elsevier Inc. All rights reserved.

CELLULAR SENESCENCE IN THE AGING KIDNEY

The expression of senescence markers has been shown to correlate well with renal aging. Numerous mechanisms of injury contribute to age-related organ dysfunction, including increased oxygen radicals and fibrogenic mediators, mitochondrial injury, and loss of telomeres (**Fig. 1**).[2] The Klotho gene, which is expressed in the distal convoluted tubules of the kidneys, is thought to be involved in the regulation of human aging.[3] Its antiaging effect through inhibition of the insulin/insulin growth factor-1 (IGF-1) pathway is associated with increased resistance to oxidative stress. In the pathogenesis of renal senescence, the downregulation of the Klotho gene increases the susceptibility to oxidant stress via stimulation of the IGF-1 pathway.[4] Increased oxidant stress in turn causes downregulation of the Klotho gene and also leads to activation of the angiotensin II pathway, which incites transcription of transforming growth factor B1 (TGF-B1). In addition, oxidative stress leads to shortening of telomeres by inhibition of telomerase and accumulation of malignant mitochondria in cells caused by activation of target of rapamycin (TOR).[5]

ANATOMIC CHANGES

Several structural and histologic changes occur with aging (**Table 1**), leading to glomerulosclerosis, increased arteriosclerosis, medial hypertrophy, and arteriolar hyalinosis.[6,7] There is also increased tubular atrophy with surrounding areas of interstitial fibrosis. This constellation of findings constitute nephrosclerosis, which increased progressively with age, 2.7% for people aged 18 to 29 years, 16% for 30 to 39 years, 28% for 40 to 49 years, 44% for 50 to 59 years, 58% for 60 to 69 years, and 73% for 70 to 77 years.[8] An age-related decline in GFR was not explained by these histologic changes occurring with normal aging.

Renal Mass

Renal mass reaches about 400 g in the fourth decade of life, after which it declines gradually to about 300 g by the ninth decade.[9] Loss of renal mass is mainly cortical,

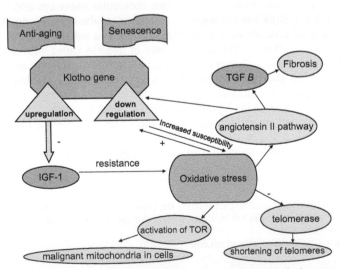

Fig. 1. Factors involved in Cellular Senescence. IGF-1, insulin growth factor-1; TGF, transforming growth factor; TOR, target of rapamycin.

Table 1
Histologic changes in the aging kidney

Glomerulus	Glomerulosclerosis Thickening of the basement membrane Increase in mesangial matrix
Tubulointerstitium	Tubulointerstitial fibrosis Decrease in tubular number Decrease in tubular volume and length
Vascular	Arteriosclerosis Hyaline deposition Aglomerulus arteriole

with relative sparing of the medulla, leading to thinning of the renal cortical parenchyma. Imaging studies that exclude persons with comorbidities show less decline in kidney volume with age.[10] Factors other than age seem to be more strongly correlated with kidney volume, including gender, body surface area, and GFR.[11]

Although kidney weight declines with age, there is no evidence of age-dependent decline in kidney volume when analyzed by computed tomography imaging. The reason for the unaltered kidney volume may be the compensatory hypertrophy of unaffected nephrons in response to the significant nephron loss caused by glomerulosclerosis and tubular atrophy.[12]

On gross examination, the senescent kidneys are symmetrically contracted with a finely granular texture of the subcapsular surface.

Glomerular Structural Changes

Glomerular shape changes with age. The spherical glomerulus in the fetal kidney develops lobular indentations as it matures, which tend to diminish with aging. Also, the length of the glomerular tuft perimeter decreases relative to the total area with age.

Various studies have reported discrepant findings regarding changes in glomerular size with aging. Although glomerular number decreases, studies differ on the size of the remaining glomeruli.[13] It is likely that both an increase in the proportion of small sclerosed glomeruli and an increase in the size of functional glomeruli occur with age.[14] Functional glomeruli often show an increase in the overall tuft cross-sectional area and thickened glomerular basement membrane. The glomerular basement membrane undergoes progressive folding, then thickening, and eventually condenses into hyaline material with glomerular tuft collapse.

Many glomerular changes noted with age share features similar to many renal conditions. Glomerular sclerosis is a nonspecific end-stage morphologic change that results from a wide range of insults, including ischemia. Glomerulosclerosis is associated with increased glomerular basement membrane and an increase in the mesangial matrix volume, which is likely a consequence of alteration in the balance between formation and breakdown of the extracellular matrix in the glomerulus.

In addition to glomerular size, glomerular density is an important surrogate of the average nephron size. Glomerular density is the number of glomeruli per area of cortex, and inversely correlates with glomerular size. In biopsy samples in which sclerotic glomeruli are less than 10%, a decrease in glomerular density is noted, which is consistent with increased size of glomeruli and tubules with aging. However, in samples in which there are more that 10% sclerotic glomeruli, glomerular density is noted to increase with increased age, consistent with the higher proportion of small sclerotic glomeruli and more tubular atrophy.[15]

The age-related findings on light microscopy of kidney biopsies include an increased proportion of globally sclerotic glomeruli, which has an ischemic appearance with tuft collapse and intracapsular fibrosis. It has been shown that living kidney donors have increased prevalence of glomerulosclerosis on renal biopsy varying with age: 19% in ages 18 to 29 years, 47% in ages 40 to 49 years, and up to 82% in ages 70 to 77 years.

Different cells within the glomeruli are also affected by aging. Age-related glomerular expansion is associated with significant mesangial expansion.[16] Mesangial cells and endothelial cells have been shown to increase in number till the age of 50 years, after which a decline is noted. The ratio of the number of glomerular mesangial cells to enlarged glomerular volume is therefore initially maintained. In contrast, podocytes do not increase in number but do exhibit hypertrophy in association with glomerular hypertrophy.

Tubulointerstitial Changes

The noted decrease in kidney size with age is thought to be a result of not only loss of glomeruli but also to be caused by tubulointerstitial changes that include infarction, scarring, and fibrosis. Tubulointerstitial fibrosis in aging is an active process associated with interstitial inflammation and fibroblast activation. The infiltrating interstitial cells consist of myofibroblasts and macrophages, with increased immunostaining for the adhesive proteins osteopontin and intercellular adhesion molecule 1, and collagen IV deposition.

Simple cysts of the kidney are also more common with older age.[17] The distal renal tubules develop diverticula that increase in number with increasing age. These diverticula in distal and collecting tubules may be precursors of simple cysts. Although tubular number is known to decrease with age, changes in tubular morphology have also been noted, including a decrease in tubule volume and length and increased tubular atrophy.[18]

Changes that have been described in the extracellular matrix include collagen alterations. Experimental models of the aging kidney showed increased collagen deposits in association with increased expression of fibrosis-related genes, including fibronectin and TGF-B.[19,20]

Vascular Changes

The blood vessel changes that occur in aging play a major role in renal damage, resulting in renal blood flow decrease with increasing age. It is thought that there are changes in both vascular responsiveness and autoregulation.[21] The intrarenal arterial changes that occur with age, which include arteriosclerosis and intimal and medial hypertrophy, are noted to be more prominent with diabetes or hypertension.[22,23] The arcuate arteries become more angulated and irregular with aging, and there is increased tortuosity and spiraling of the interlobar vessels. In the arterioles, hyaline deposits within the vessel walls lead to obliteration of the lumen, and are associated with sclerotic glomeruli mainly in the cortex. With aging, a continuous channel develops between the afferent and efferent arterioles, where blood is shunted to the medullary area, leading to an aglomerulus arteriole and resulting in sclerotic glomeruli.

In a classic study of renal vascular responses in normal aging men, Hollenberg and colleagues[24] found that the vasodilatory response to acetylcholine or to an acute sodium load was impaired with aging. In contrast, the vasoconstrictive response to angiotensin was not altered with aging, consistent with a fixed anatomic lesion of blood vessels.

PHYSIOLOGIC CHANGES
Mediators of Age-related Physiologic Changes

There are several physiologic changes that occur in the aging kidney (**Box 1**). With aging, there is a propensity toward an increased sensitivity to vasoconstrictor stimuli and reduced vasodilatory response. Sclerosis occurs via tissue mediators such as angiotensin II, TGF-B, advanced glycation end products, and oxidative stress.[25,26] The increased oxidative stress that accompanies aging results in endothelial cell dysfunction and changes in vasoactive mediators.

There is decreased renin production and release with aging, and the total aldosterone level consequently decreases.[27] Although the systemic renin-angiotensin system (RAS) is suppressed in aging, the intrarenal RAS may not be equivalently suppressed. Angiotensin II has numerous effects on the kidney that affect filtration pressure and proximal tubular sodium and water transport.[28,29] It also affects tubular and glomerular growth, nitric oxide (NO) synthesis, oxidative stress, inflammation, cell migration, apoptosis, and protein accumulation in the extracellular matrix.[30] All these factors can affect renal glomerulosclerosis and tubulointerstitial fibrosis. Regression of age-related glomerular and vascular sclerosis was noted in rats treated with angiotensin II antagonists.[31]

The balance of vasoconstrictor and vasodilatory responsiveness plays an important part in the kidney's response to acute injury. NO plays a diverse role in renal vasculature and cell growth and has a protective effect. There is a notable decrease in NO level with aging, which is thought to lead to increased renal vasoconstriction and sodium retention, as well as increased matrix production and mesangial fibrosis.[32] Levels of NO are higher in the medullary region and are reduced in the renal cortex, which may contribute to reduced perfusion in the elderly.[33]

Sex hormones are also thought to play a role in age-related changes in the RAS and NO systems. Estrogen seems to have a protective effect, because 17B-estradiol decreases tissue levels and activity of angiotensin II and angiotensin-converting enzyme. Men may be at increased risk of renal dysfunction because of the negative effects of androgens, which tend to increase RAS activity.[34] Androgens also inhibit age-related increase in metalloproteinases, which help prevent matrix expansion, resulting in increased fibrosis and mesangial matrix production.

GFR

The GFR is low at birth, reaches adult levels by the second year of life, and is maintained at 140 mL/min/1.73 m^2 until the fourth decade of life when the decline is about 8 mL/min/1.73 m^2 per decade.[35] When accurate creatinine clearances are performed, there is clear evidence for a reduction in mean creatinine clearance per age group despite no difference in serum creatinine. The inclusion of age and gender in all the serum creatinine–based equations is to account for an anticipated

---

Box 1
Functional changes in the aging kidney

Decrease in GFR by 8 mL/min/1.73 m^2 per decade after age 30 years

Decrease in renal blood flow

Increase in glomerular basement membrane permeability

Decreased ability to dilute and concentrate urine

Decreased ability to excrete acid load

endogenous decline in creatinine production rate with age caused by loss of lean body mass.[36]

The functional reserve of the kidney, defined as the acute increase in basal GFR by 20% after an infusion of amino acids, was around 15% in healthy elderly volunteers and it was maintained until the age of 80 years.[37] This increase in functional reserve was not accompanied by an increase of effective renal blood flow or a significant decrease in renal vascular resistance, which suggests that the increase in renal reserve in the elderly was not related to vasodilatation, as is commonly found in young individuals.

The rate of decline in renal function with aging is thought to be greatly influenced by comorbidities including hypertension and cardiovascular disease. One study that dissociated the renal functional changes accompanying normal senescence from diseases of aging concerned Kuna Indians, an island-dwelling indigenous population that was free of cardiovascular disease and hypertension.[38] Both the GFR and renal plasma flow declined with age in the Kuna Indians. Furthermore, in living donor biopsy series, GFR declined with aging independently of nephrosclerosis, raising the question of other pathologic changes in the kidney and extrarenal factors contributing to the decline in GFR.[39]

Renal Plasma Flow

Renal blood flow is maintained at 600 mL/min until approximately the fourth decade, and then declines by about 10% per decade.[40] Xenon washout studies have shown that there is a progressive decline in renal blood flow per unit kidney mass. This reduction is therefore not entirely caused by loss of renal mass. The decrease in renal blood flow is most profound in the renal cortex. The reduction in renal plasma blood flow is greater than the decrease in GFR, resulting in increased filtration fraction in elderly persons.[41] The decline in renal plasma flow tends to be greater in men than in women. A possible explanation for the decreased renal blood flow may be that it is caused by an imbalance and alterations in the responsiveness of vasoactive substances.

Capillary Permeability and Proteinuria

Animal studies have shown an increase in glomerular basement membrane permeability, leading to an increase in urinary excretion of proteins.[42] Even in the absence of diabetes, hypertension, and chronic kidney disease, there is increased incidence of both microalbuminuria and overt proteinuria with advanced age. The decreased sulfation of the glomerular basement membrane glycoaminoglycans may account for the increased permeability of the glomerular basement membrane to macromolecules.[43]

Osmoregulation/Sodium and Water Handling

Elderly persons are not able to dilute or concentrate their urine as well as younger healthy individuals, and are consequently more prone to water disorders and volume depletion. The ability to generate free water depends on several factors, which include adequate delivery of solute to the diluting region as a result of sufficient renal perfusion and GFR, a functional intact distal diluting site, and suppression of antidiuretic hormone (ADH) to avoid water reabsorption in the collecting duct.[44] The age-related decline in GFR is an important factor in the aged kidney's diluting capacity. Studies of the diluting capacity of the aged kidney found that minimal urine osmolality in men with a mean age of 31 years was 52 mOsm/kg and 92 mOsm/kg in the older men with a mean age of 84 years after water loading.[45] The free-water clearance was lowest in the oldest group, but the results were the same when free-water clearance was expressed as milliliters per minute of GFR, which implies that the defect in diluting capacity is a function of age-related reduction in GFR.

Studies in aged rats with normal ADH receptors suggest that the downregulation of V2 receptors in renal tubules results in the functional impairment of renal concentrating ability. Water reabsorption in the collecting duct is also thought to be further affected by the lower abundance of aquaporins 2 and 3 in aged rats.[46] Compared with younger age groups undergoing a 12-hour water deprivation test in the Baltimore longitudinal study, subjects aged 60 to 79 years had a 20% lower maximal urine osmolality, 100% increase in minimal urine flow rate, and a 50% decrease in the ability to conserve solutes. This effect of age persisted after correction for age-related decrease in GFR.[47] In an older study of age-related changes in renal concentrating capacity following a 24-hour water deprivation test, the maximal attainable urine specific gravity declined from 1.030 at 40 years to 1.023 at 89 years.[48] The clinical significance of diminished water-conserving capacity may not be consequential until access to free water becomes limited in the elderly.[49]

In the elderly, the capacity to conserve sodium in response to reduced sodium intake is reduced. Restriction in intake to 10 mEq per day resulted in a half-time reduction of urinary sodium of 17.6 hours in young individuals and 30.9 hours in elderly participants.[50] Also, elderly individuals are more likely to have an exaggerated natriuresis after a water load. The exact mechanism has not been elucidated but reduction in the number of functioning nephrons along with reduced aldosterone secretion is thought to play a role.

In the elderly, the fractional proximal sodium reabsorption is significantly higher than it is in young individuals, but this increase is offset by the lower distal fractional reabsorption of sodium.[51] Given the described age-related decrease in renal blood flow and GFR, sodium retention is favored, and the elderly are prone to fluid volume expansion when challenged with a sodium load. An impaired response to angiotensin II is one possible mechanism. Elderly individuals also seem to have more sodium excretion at night, suggesting an impaired circadian variation.

Electrolyte and Acid-Base Changes

Elderly people are capable of secreting an acid load and maintain normal serum bicarbonate levels and an appropriate urine pH on a 70-g protein diet.[52] However, senescent kidneys challenged with an acute acid load do not increase acid excretion and lower urinary pH to the degree that younger kidneys do. The maximum capacity to generate ammonia seems to be reduced in the elderly. In addition, there is a reduction in the abundance of the major urea transporter in the inner medullary collecting duct, which could result in decreased urea reabsorption and thus cause a reduction in inner medullary osmolality.[1]

Potassium handling in aging kidneys is also affected by aging. Impaired potassium secretion, which is directly associated with disorders in sodium reabsorption, may occur in aging kidneys because of tubular atrophy and tubular interstitial scarring. Hyporeninemic hypoaldosteronism and volume depletion–related suppression of water and sodium delivery into the distal nephron is also associated with potassium secretion disorders in aging kidneys.[53,54]

REFERENCES

1. Lindeman RD, Tobin J, Shock NW. Longitudinal studies on the rate of decline in renal function with age. J Am Geriatr Soc 1985;33:278–85.

2. Perico N, Remuzzi G, Benigni A. Aging and the kidney. Curr Opin Nephrol Hypertens 2011;20:312–7.
3. Kanasaki K, Kitada M, Koya D. Pathophysiology of the aging kidney and therapeutic interventions. Hypertens Res 2012;35:1121–8.
4. Yang H, Fogo A. Cell senescence in the aging kidney. J Am Soc Nephrol 2010; 21:1436–9.
5. Zhou X, Saxena R, Liu Z, et al. Renal senescence in 2008: progress and challenges. Int Urol Nephrol 2008;40:823–39.
6. Martin JE, Sheaff MT. Renal ageing. J Pathol 2007;211:198–205.
7. Glassock R, Rule A. The implications of anatomic and functional changes in the aging kidney: with an emphasis on the glomeruli. Kidney Int 2010;80:270–7.
8. Ruler AD, Amer H, Cornell LD, et al. The association between age and nephrosclerosis on renal biopsy among healthy adults. Ann Intern Med 2010;152: 561–7.
9. McLachlan M, Wasserman P. Changes in the size and distensibility of the aging kidney. Br J Radiol 1981;54:488–91.
10. Rao UV, Wagner HN Jr. Normal weights of human organs. Radiology 1972;102: 337–9.
11. Kasiske BL, Umen AJ. The influence of age, sex, race and body habitus on kidney weight in humans. Arch Pathol Lab Med 1986;110:55–60.
12. Goyal VK. Changes with age in the human kidney. Exp Gerontol 1982;17: 321–31.
13. Hoy WE, Douglas-Denton RN, Highson MD, et al. A stereological study of glomerular number and volume: preliminary findings in a multiracial study of kidneys at autopsy. Kidney Int Suppl 2003;63:S31–7.
14. Abdi R, Slakey D, Kittur D. Heterogeneity of glomerular size in normal donor kidneys: impact of race. Am J Kidney Dis 1998;32:43–6.
15. Rule AD, Semret MH, Amer H, et al. Association of kidney function and metabolic risk factors with density of glomeruli on renal biopsy samples from living donors. Mayo Clin Proc 2011;86:282–90.
16. Anderson S, Brenner BM. Effects of aging on the renal glomerulus. Am J Med 1986;80(3):435–42.
17. Lauks SP Jr, McClachlan MS. Aging and simple cysts of the kidney. Br J Radiol 1981;54(637):12–4.
18. Lindeman RD, Goldman R. Anatomic and physiologic age changes in the kidney. Exp Gerontol 1986;21(4–5):379–406.
19. Takizawa T, Takasaki I, Shionoiri H, et al. Progression of glomerulosclerosis, renal hypertrophy, and an increased expression of fibronectin in the renal cortex associated with aging and salt-induced hypertension in Dahl salt-sensitive rats. Life Sci 1997;61(16):1553–8.
20. Gagliano N, Arioso B, Santanbrogio B, et al. Age-dependent expression of fibrosis-related genes and collagen deposition in rat kidney cortex. J Gerontol A Biol Sci Med Sci 2000;55(8):365–72.
21. McDonald RK, Solomon DH, Shock NW. Aging as a factor in the renal hemodynamic changes induced by a standard pyrogen. J Clin Invest 1951;5: 457–62.
22. Kubo M, Kyiohara Y, Kato I, et al. Risk factors of renal glomerular and vascular changes in an autopsy based population survey: the Hisayama study. Kidney Int 2003;63:1508–15.
23. McLachlan MS, Guthrie JC, Anderson CK, et al. Vascular and glomerular changes in the ageing kidney. J Pathol 1977;121:65–78.

24. Hollenberg NK, Adams DF, Solomon HS, et al. Senescence and the renal vasculature in normal man. Circ Res 1974;34:309–16.
25. Thomas MC, Tikellis C, Burns WM, et al. Interactions between renin angiotensin system and advanced glycation in the kidney. J Am Soc Nephrol 2005;16: 2976–84.
26. Ruiz-Torres MP, Bosch RJ, O'Valle F, et al. Age-related increase in expression of TGF-beta1 in the rat kidney: relationship to morphologic changes. J Am Soc Nephrol 1998;9:782–91.
27. Weidmann P, De Myttenaere-Bursztein S, Maxwell MH, et al. Effect of aging on plasma renin and aldosterone in normal man. Kidney Int 1975;8:325–33.
28. Cogan MG. Angiotensin II: a powerful controller of sodium transport in the early proximal tubule. Hypertension 1990;15:451–8.
29. Norman JT. The role of angiotensin II in renal growth. Ren Physiol Biochem 1991; 14:175–85.
30. Choudhury D, Levi M. Kidney aging–inevitable or preventable. Nat Rev Nephrol 2011;7:706–17.
31. Ma LJ, Nakamura S, Aldigier AC, et al. Regression of glomerulosclerosis with high-dose angiotensin inhibition is linked to decreased plasminogen activator inhibitor-1. J Am Soc Nephrol 2005;16:966–76.
32. Weinstein J, Anderson S. The aging kidney: physiological changes. Adv Chronic Kidney Dis 2010;17(4):302–7.
33. Llorens S, Fernandez AP, Nava E. Cardiovascular and renal alterations on the nitric oxide pathway in spontaneous hypertension and ageing. Clin Hemorheol Microcirc 2007;37:149–56.
34. Fortepiani LA, Yanes L, Zhang H, et al. Role of androgens in mediating renal injury in aging SHR. Hypertension 2003;42:952–5.
35. Rowe JW, Andres RA, Tobin JD, et al. The effect of age on creatinine clearance in man: a cross-sectional and longitudinal study. J Gerontol 1976;311:155–63.
36. Epstein M. Aging and the kidney. J Am Soc Nephrol 1996;7:1106–22.
37. Fliser D, Zeler M, Nowack R, et al. Renal function reserve in healthy elderly subjects. J Am Soc Nephrol 1993;3:1371–7.
38. Hollenberg NK, Rivera A, Meinking A, et al. Age, renal perfusion and function in island dwelling indigenous Kuna Americans of Panama. Nephron 1999;82:131–8.
39. Rule AD, Cornell LD, Poggio ED. Senile nephrosclerosis–does it explain the decline in glomerular filtration rate with aging? Nephron Physiol 2011; 119(Suppl 1):6–11.
40. Davies DF, Shock NW. Age changes in glomerular filtration, effective renal plasma flow and tubular excretory capacity in adult males. J Clin Invest 1950; 29:496–506.
41. Davies DF, Shock NW. Renal blood flow. J Clin Invest 1950;29:496–500.
42. Bolton WK, Benton FR, Maclay JG, et al. Spontaneous glomerular sclerosis in aging Sprague-Dawley rats. Am J Pathol 1976;85:227–302.
43. Cohen MP, Ku L. Age-related changes in sulfation of basement membrane glycosaminoglycans. Exp Gerontol 1976;18:447–50.
44. Schalekamp MA, Krauss XH, Schalekamp-Kuyken MP, et al. Studies on the mechanism of hypernatriuresis in essential hypertension in relation to measurement of plasma renin concentration, body fluid compartment and renal function. Clin Sci 1971;41:219–31.
45. Lindeman RD, Lee DT, Yiegst MJ, et al. Influence of age, renal disease, hypertension, diuretics and calcium on the antidiuretic responses to suboptimal infusions of vasopressin. J Lab Clin Med 1966;68:202–23.

46. Preisser L, Teillet L, Aliotti S, et al. Downregulation of aquaporin-2 and -3 in aging kidney is independent of V(2) vasopressin receptor. Am J Physiol Renal Physiol 2000;279:F144–52.
47. Rowe JW, Shock NW, DeFronzo RA. The influence of age on renal response to water deprivation in man. Nephron 1976;17:270–8.
48. Lindeman RD, Van Burenc HC, Raisz LG. Osmolar renal concentrating ability in healthy young men and hospitalized patients without renal disease. N Engl J Med 1960;262:1306–9.
49. Faubert PF, Porush JG. Renal disease in the elderly. 2nd edition. New York: Marcel Dekker; 1998. p. 15–128.
50. Epstein M, Hollenberg NK. Age as a determinant of renal sodium conservation in normal man. J Lab Clin Med 1976;87:411–7.
51. Miller M. Hormonal aspects of fluid and sodium balance in the elderly. Endocrinol Metab Clin North Am 1995;24:233–53.
52. Wagner EA, Falciglia GA, Amlal H, et al. Short-term exposure to a high-protein diet differentially affects glomerular filtration rate but not acid-base balance in older compared to younger adults. J Am Diet Assoc 2007;107:1404–8.
53. Perez GO, Lespier L, Jacobi J. Hyporeninemia and hypoaldosteronism in diabetes mellitus. Arch Intern Med 1977;137:852–5.
54. Phelps KR, Lieberman RL, Oh MS, et al. Pathophysiology of the syndrome of hyporeninemic hypoaldosteronism. Metabolism 1980;29:186–99.

Acute Kidney Injury in the Elderly

Mitchell H. Rosner, MD

KEYWORDS

- Elderly • Acute kidney injury • Dialysis • Outcome

KEY POINTS

- Acute kidney injury (AKI) is a disease of the elderly with an increasing incidence over the past decade.
- Specific causes of AKI such as acute tubular necrosis and obstructive nephropathy are more commonly seen in the elderly population.
- AKI is associated with a significant increase in mortality and morbidity, and preventive strategies are required to mitigate risk.
- Although many elderly patients with AKI may have poor outcomes, age alone should not be used as a determinant for care, as many patients will have a good outcome.
- Patients surviving AKI are often left with chronic kidney disease, and will need close follow-up by a nephrologist.

INTRODUCTION

Acute kidney injury (AKI) is a common and serious event, most often complicating hospitalization for serious illness.[1] In its most severe form (requiring dialysis support), AKI is associated with a very high rate of mortality and morbidity both in the index hospital stay and after discharge.[2–4] Important recent data demonstrate that from 2000 to 2009 the incidence of dialysis-requiring AKI increased from 222 to 533 cases per million person-years; an average increase of 10% per year.[5] An important factor driving this increase in AKI over the past decade is the older age of the population, which serves as an independent risk factor for the development of AKI. For instance, hospitalized patients with dialysis-requiring AKI are older than their counterparts without dialysis-requiring AKI (63.4 vs 47.6 years).[5]

It is not hard to hypothesize why elderly patients have an increased risk for AKI. These patients have a large number of comorbid conditions accumulated over their life span that can lead to chronic kidney disease (CKD), they are exposed to multiple potentially nephrotoxic medications and invasive procedures, and they have specific

Disclosure: The author has no relevant financial relationships to disclose.
Division of Nephrology, University of Virginia Health System, Box 800133 HSC, Charlottesville, VA 22908, USA
E-mail address: MHR9R@hscmail.mcc.virginia.edu

structural, functional, and molecular changes in their kidneys that decrease renal reserve and increase susceptibility to severe damage when faced with an insult. The knowledge gained in a deeper understanding of these risks associated with AKI in the elderly patient should be used to develop preventive and protective strategies that decrease the likelihood of dialysis-requiring AKI and also hasten resolution of AKI when it cannot be avoided. This review focuses on the epidemiology, risk and susceptibility factors, prevention, and therapy for AKI in this vulnerable patient group.

EPIDEMIOLOGY

Although studies describing the incidence of AKI in this population are difficult to compare because the definitions of AKI vary dramatically from study to study, it is clear that the elderly are at the very highest risk for the development of AKI. One could even argue that AKI is largely a disease of the elderly.

- Feest and colleagues[6] demonstrated that there is a 3- to 8-fold, progressive, age-dependent increase in the frequency of community-acquired AKI in patients older than 60 years.
- Over the past 25 years, the mean age of patients with AKI has increased by at least 5 years and perhaps as much as 15 years.[7]
- Groeneveld and colleagues[8] demonstrated that the age-related yearly incidence of AKI rose from 17 per million in adults younger than 50 years to 949 per million in the 80- to 89-year-old age group.
- A 9-year, prospective study in Madrid, Spain demonstrated a 3.5-fold greater incidence of AKI in patients older than 70 years.[9]
- Ali and colleagues[10] demonstrated that the average age of patients with AKI in a large European cohort was 76 years. However, the average age of those patients with acute on chronic renal failure was 80.5 years, and this group had a much higher risk for adverse outcomes.[10]
- Hsu and colleagues[3] most recently also demonstrated that not only were elderly patients at higher risk for the most severe form of AKI (that requiring dialysis) in comparison with younger patients, but that over time the incidence of AKI in the elderly is increasing more rapidly than in younger cohorts (**Fig. 1**).

The outcomes for elderly patients who develop dialysis-requiring AKI are uniformly poor, with reported mortality rates ranging from 31% to 80% (with the highest mortality seen in patients requiring dialysis).[11] In part, the wide variation in these mortality rates is due to study inclusion criteria, whether mortality related to intensive care unit (ICU) rather than hospital discharge was studied, and definitions for advanced age. For example:

- The BEST Kidney study showed that advanced age was independently associated with increased hospital mortality in patients with AKI.[12]
- Bagshaw and colleagues[13] also found an association between advanced age and higher 1-year mortality in ICU patients with severe AKI.

In those patients who survive their episode of AKI, an important consideration is whether recovery of renal function also occurs, and what the long-term burden of renal injury may be. In a meta-analysis, Schmitt and colleagues found that patients older than 65 years had significantly worse renal recovery rates than younger patients (31.3% of surviving elderly patients did not recover kidney function compared with 26% of younger patients).[14] Other studies have also demonstrated that the rates of renal recovery after AKI are lower in the elderly.[15,16] Thus, in those elderly patients

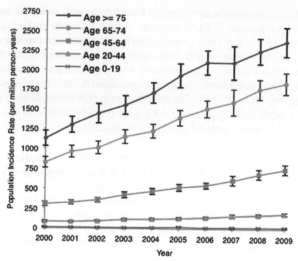

Fig. 1. Population incidence of dialysis-requiring acute kidney injury in the United States from 2000 to 2009. (*Reprinted from* Hsu RK, McCulloch CE, Dudley RA, et al. Temporal changes in incidence of dialysis-requiring AKI. J Am Soc Nephrol 2013;24(1):37–42; with permission.)

who develop dialysis-requiring AKI the likelihood of renal recovery is lower, leaving patients with the burden of significant CKD and possibly end-stage renal disease (ESRD).

WHAT ACCOUNTS FOR THE INCREASED SUSCEPTIBILITY OF THE ELDERLY TO AKI?

Overall, the factors that increase the risk of AKI in the elderly patient can be divided into several main categories:

1. *Comorbid conditions.* The incidence of comorbid conditions that increase the risk for AKI dramatically increases with age. Hypertension, diabetes mellitus, atherosclerosis, and heart failure are all conditions more commonly encountered in older individuals, and all can directly or indirectly increase the risk for AKI. For instance, atherosclerosis and hypertension impair the autoregulatory capacity of the kidney to maintain perfusion in the setting of hypotension. Thus, modest decreases in systemic blood pressure may be associated with significant ischemic damage to the kidney.[17] More directly, these conditions are associated with the development of glomerulosclerosis and CKD as well as the use of medications (such as angiotensin-converting enzyme inhibitors and angiotensin receptor blockers) that increase the risk of AKI in certain settings.[18] These conditions may also lead to the need for invasive procedures such as cardiovascular surgery and percutaneous revascularization, which are associated with a high risk for AKI. Another comorbid condition more commonly seen in the elderly is prostatic disease, which when severe can lead to urinary tract obstruction. The important role of prostatic disease in causing AKI is highlighted by that fact that 35% of AKI cases in patients aged 80 to 89 years were accounted for by this cause in one study.[6]
2. *Chronic kidney disease.* In nearly all studies assessing the risk for AKI, baseline kidney function stands out as one of the most important factors affecting risk, with those with the lowest baseline glomerular filtration rate (GFR) having the highest risk.[17] Data from the National Health and Nutrition Examination Survey (NHANES)

suggest that CKD prevalence is highest in the elderly, with a 38% prevalence rate in those older than 65 years.[19] Furthermore, elderly patients with CKD also have a high prevalence of the aforementioned conditions that increase the risk for AKI.[20] For instance, in the Kidney Early Evaluation Program (KEEP) for patients older than 65 years, 89% had hypertension and 41% had diabetes mellitus.[20]

3. *Polypharmacy.* Elderly patients are often prescribed a large number of medications with an associated increased risk for adverse drug reactions (ADRs). In the ICU, the most frequent ADR is drug-induced AKI, and cardiovascular drugs are the most frequent culprits.[21] Thus, careful review of medications and minimization of drug-drug interactions is critically important in this population. Whenever possible, dosing should be based either on drug levels or titration to clinical effect. It is also important to note that the aging kidney is less able to clear pharmacologic agents and thus toxic levels may occur more often.

4. *Structural, functional, and hemodynamic changes in the kidney associated with aging.* Numerous age-related changes may affect the ability of the kidney to withstand an injurious insult. These factors all make it more likely that a given insult may not be able to be compensated for and, thus, will result in larger and more significant damage.
   a. Structural changes
      i. Total renal mass declines with age[22]
      ii. The number of functioning glomeruli decreases with age[23]
   b. Functional changes
      i. Variable decline in GFR with age[24]
      ii. A change in sodium homeostasis results in an impaired ability to concentrate urine, and increases the risk of volume depletion in the elderly[25]
   c. Hemodynamic changes
      i. Decreased renal blood flow and decreased blood flow reserve[26]
      ii. Increased renal vascular resistance[27]
      iii. Impaired renal vasodilatation and exaggerated renal vasoconstriction[28]
      iv. Impaired autoregulation[28]
      v. Impaired nitric oxide production[29]

5. *Cellular and molecular changes in the aging kidney that increase the risk for AKI.* Aging is associated with cellular changes that make renal tubular cells more vulnerable to insults. These changes include:
   a. Increased oxidative stress and impaired oxidative stress defenses[30]
   b. Decreased cellular proliferation rates and increased expression of genes inhibiting cellular proliferation[31]
   c. Increased expression of senescent-related genes[32]

ETIOLOGY OF AKI IN THE ELDERLY

The causes of AKI in the elderly patient span the typical causes seen in other populations, with some notable differences (**Box 1**). In general, elderly patients with AKI may have suffered from multiple insults as well as having a higher incidence of prerenal, nephrotoxic, and obstructive causes.

- Prerenal AKI in some series accounts for nearly one-third of AKI causes.[33] AKI in this circumstance is due to decreased renal perfusion from any cause such as heart failure or depletion of effective circulating volume. Elderly patients are more prone to the development of volume depletion and dehydration.[34] In part, this is due to impairment in renal concentrating ability but also to the use of diuretics, impaired thirst sensation and, in some cases, restricted ability

Box 1
Causes of acute kidney injury

- Prerenal
  - Loss of fluids due to vomiting, diarrhea, diuretics, hyperglycemia
  - Insufficient fluid replacement or access in setting of continued fluid loss
  - Redistribution of intravascular volume ("third-spacing")
  - Decreased cardiac output of any etiology (heart failure, valvular disease, pericardial disease, ischemia, arrhythmias)
  - Use of medications that impair renal autoregulation and intrarenal hemodynamics
    - Nonsteroidal anti-inflammatory medications
    - Angiotensin-converting enzyme inhibitors
    - Angiotensin receptor blockers
    - Calcineurin inhibitors
  - Hypercalcemia (usually associated with malignancy)
- Renal (intrinsic)
  - ATN (ischemic [sepsis] or nephrotoxic)
  - Vascular etiology (atheroembolic, large-vessel vasculitis, renal artery obstruction)
  - Rapidly progressive glomerulonephritis (most often antineutrophil cytoplasmic antibody–positive)
  - Acute interstitial nephritis (usually allergic related to medications)
- Postrenal (obstructive)
  - Upper tract
    - Bilateral nephrolithiasis or nephrolithiasis in a single kidney
    - Pelvic neoplasms and lymphoma
    - Retroperitoneal disease (fibrosis, neoplasms, adenopathy, hematoma)
    - Prior history of radiation therapy
  - Lower tract
    - Prostatic disease (malignancy or hypertrophy)
    - Pelvic malignancies
    - Bladder carcinoma
    - Nephrolithiasis
    - Blood clots
    - Urethral strictures (due to past trauma or disease)
    - Neurogenic bladder

to access fluids. A common scenario is a bedridden nursing home resident who develops a diarrheal illness with the inability to increase oral intake to match stool-volume losses. These patients often present with severe hypernatremia and AKI. It is also important to be aware that the traditional signs of volume depletion may be difficult to discern in the elderly patient. For example, due to the age-related declines in tubular sodium handling or the use of diuretics, the fractional excretion of sodium may be elevated despite volume depletion.

In many cases, therefore, a judicious trial of intravenous fluids may be warranted.

- Intrarenal causes of AKI include a heterogeneous group of disorders that can be subgrouped according to the anatomic compartment of the kidney that is injured (ie, the vasculature, tubules, interstitium, or glomeruli).
  1. Vasculature. Acute obstruction of the renal vasculature is an uncommon cause of AKI, but can be seen in the elderly patient undergoing a vascular procedure leading to cholesterol embolization. A more common occurrence is AKI caused by changes in intrarenal hemodynamics that disturb the normal autoregulatory capacity of the kidney to maintain GFR over a wide range of blood pressure. In the elderly patient, drugs that impair normal circulatory homeostatic mechanisms such as angiotensin-converting enzyme inhibitors, angiotensin receptor blockers, or nonsteroidal anti-inflammatory drugs can lead to significant decreases in GFR, especially in states where renal perfusion may be marginal (such as cirrhosis, heart failure, or volume depletion).
  2. Acute tubular necrosis (ATN). In most series, ATN is the most common cause of AKI in the elderly.[33,35]
     - Nephrotoxic causes include medications such as aminoglycosides, radiocontrast material, and chemotherapeutic agents. Pigments attributable to hemolysis or rhabdomyolysis are less common offenders.
     - Ischemia, when prolonged and severe, can result in tubular injury. Major causes include sepsis, severe and prolonged volume depletion, and major surgical procedures (most commonly involving the cardiovascular system).
  3. Acute interstitial nephritis (AIN). Data on incidence of AIN in the elderly is lacking. However, given the large number of medications that are prescribed to this group of patients, clinicians must always consider this as a possible diagnosis. Classically the presence of urine eosinophils was thought to be diagnostic of AIN, but this finding has a very low sensitivity and is not specific for this diagnosis.[36] Recently, proton-pump inhibitors have been implicated as a cause of AIN.[37]
  4. Glomerulonephritis. A rapidly progressive glomerulonephritis could present as AKI, typically with manifestations in other organ systems. Clinicians should consider this possibility when the urinalysis displays dysmorphic red blood cells, red blood cell casts, and proteinuria. In the elderly, the most common cause of this presentation would be antineutrophil cytoplasmic antibody (ANCA)-associated diseases, most commonly p-ANCA or positive antimyeloperoxidase.[38] A renal biopsy should be pursued when a rapidly progressive glomerulonephritis is considered as a potential cause of AKI, as there are no age-related increases in biopsy complications.[39] Findings of significant glomerulosclerosis and tubular atrophy may temper one's enthusiasm to use high-dose immunosuppressive medications, which have a higher likelihood of morbidity in the elderly.[40]
- Postrenal causes of AKI are more commonly encountered in elderly patients, with an incidence of approximately 10%.[41,42] Common causes in the male patient include prostate disease (benign prostatic hypertrophy or prostate carcinoma) or urethral stricture; whereas in females pelvic malignancies are the primary cause. An additional cause may be neurogenic bladder associated with the use of anticholinergic medications. All elderly patients presenting with AKI require urethral catheterization as well as renal ultrasonography to assess for urinary tract obstruction.

DIAGNOSTIC WORKUP FOR AKI IN THE ELDERLY

The diagnostic workup for AKI begins with a thorough history and physical examination investigating for signs of prerenal, renal, or postrenal etiology. A thorough review of medication use, recent procedures, urine output, and signs and symptoms of systemic disease are mandatory. A renal ultrasonogram, bladder catheterization, and examination of the urinalysis are critical in arriving at a diagnosis. The finding of pigmented granular casts in the urine indicates tubular injury and ATN.[43] A potential diagnosis of glomerulonephritis is facilitated by the finding of dysmorphic red blood cells or red blood cell casts in the urine, and should prompt consideration of a kidney biopsy. White blood cells, especially eosinophils in the urine, indicate interstitial nephritis.

Urine electrolytes can also be helpful in the diagnosis of prerenal causes whereby the renal tubules remain avid for sodium and water.[44] In this case the urine sodium is low, fractional excretion of sodium is less than 1%, and the urine osmolality is elevated. An important caveat to this in the elderly patient is that many patients may have impaired sodium- and water-conserving ability or may be taking diuretics, which could lead to high urine sodium and high fractional excretion of sodium despite volume depletion. In these cases, a low fractional excretion of urea (<40%) can help indicate a prerenal etiology.[45]

LIMITATIONS OF SERUM CREATININE IN DIAGNOSING AKI IN THE ELDERLY

Serum creatinine elevations are typically used to diagnose AKI along with changes in the urine output (**Box 2**). However, this laboratory measure has significant limitations, particularly in elderly patients. Serum creatinine levels depend on the creatinine generation rate, volume of distribution, and removal rate through renal elimination. Therefore factors such as age, muscle mass, hydration status, and race may influence creatinine values. For instance, elderly patients may have decreased muscle mass and lower serum creatinine values independent of renal function.[46] Thus, a patient with a low serum creatinine value may still have AKI, and absolute creatinine values can be misleading. As an example, a serum creatinine of 1.0 mg/dL in a 45-kg 80-year-old woman may represent significantly impaired GFR, whereas this same value in a 25-year-old 70-kg man would reflect normal kidney function. Regression equations,

---

Box 2
Kidney Disease Improving Global Outcomes (KDIGO) criteria for the diagnosis of acute kidney injury

- Stage 1 AKI: 1.5–1.9 times baseline, OR $\geq$0.3 mg/dL ($\geq$26.5 μmol/L) increase in the serum creatinine, OR urine output <0.5 mL/kg per hour for 6–12 hours

- Stage 2 AKI: 2.0–2.9 times baseline increase in the serum creatinine OR urine output <0.5 mL/ kg per hour for $\geq$12 hours

- Stage 3 AKI: 3.0 times baseline increase in the serum creatinine, OR increase in serum creatinine to $\geq$4.0 mg/dL ($\geq$353.6 μmol/L), OR urine output of <0.3 mL/kg per hour for $\geq$24 hours, OR anuria for $\geq$12 hours, OR the initiation of renal replacement therapy, OR, in patients <18 years, decrease in estimated glomerular filtration rate to <35 mL/min per 1.73 m^2

Data from Clinical practice guidelines for acute kidney injury 2012. Available at: http://www. kdigo.org/clinical_practice_guidelines/AKI.php. Accessed December 16, 2012.

which translate serum creatinine values into GFR, may be helpful in this regard but have not been validated in the very elderly (age >80 years) and are only useful in steady-state conditions.[47] Caution should therefore be exercised in the diagnosis of AKI using absolute values of serum creatinine, and following serial changes in this laboratory value can be more helpful.

Sensitive urine and serum biomarkers that are more specific for the diagnosis of AKI are in development, and include biomarkers such as neutrophil gelatinase-associated lipocalin (NGAL), kidney injury marker 1, and interleukin-18.[48] These biomarkers hold promise for rapid, early detection of AKI, similar to the use of troponin in the diagnosis of cardiac ischemia.[49]

TREATMENT OF AKI IN THE ELDERLY

There are no specific therapies for AKI once it is has occurred. Thus the management of AKI is largely supportive, through maintenance of adequate renal blood flow, avoidance of further injury, and renal replacement support (if necessary). The decision to initiate renal replacement therapy (RRT) in elderly persons may be difficult and complex, given the possibility that older persons may not fare well on this aggressive, life-sustaining type of therapy and may have competing comorbid conditions that lead to a very poor overall prognosis. Hemodialysis in the elderly patient with AKI may also be poorly tolerated owing to patient-based factors such as decreased cardiovascular reserve, autonomic dysfunction, and an increased tendency toward bleeding complications. However, the few studies that have examined whether there is a survival difference between older and younger patients with severe AKI receiving RRT have not found any effect of older age on hospital survival.[42,50,51] In fact, several studies demonstrate that the mortality from AKI in elderly persons (including AKI requiring RRT) has decreased over the past several years.[52–54]

Decisions about dialysis initiation in older adults with AKI must be individualized and account for numerous factors, including the severity of illness, likelihood of meaningful physical and cognitive recovery, and wishes of the family and patient. In this regard, the recent Renal Physician Association guidelines for shared decision making in the appropriate initiation of and withdrawal from dialysis can provide a useful framework for these difficult decisions (**Box 3**).[55] In certain circumstances, a time-limited trial of dialysis for those patients with an uncertain prognosis may be warranted. However, all members of the care team and family should agree in advance on the length of the trial as well as the parameters to be assessed during and at the completion of the time-limited trial, to determine if dialysis has benefited the patient and whether dialysis should be continued.

OUTCOMES OF AKI IN THE ELDERLY

Patients with AKI may follow several trajectories after the development of the injury: (1) they may recover completely; (2) they may require permanent RRT; (3) they may partially recover and be left with CKD; or (4) they may die of their acute illness. In the past few years, new data have shed light on these various outcomes.

As discussed previously, mortality associated with AKI is directly related to the severity of the renal insult, with dialysis-requiring AKI having mortality as high as 80% in some studies.[56] Furthermore, several studies have demonstrated that older age is itself an independent risk factor for mortality in patients with AKI in the ICU.[12,57–59] Of interest, it does seem that more elderly individuals with severe AKI are surviving in the ICU, so the prevalence of long-term adverse consequences related to AKI may end up being a substantial burden in the modern era.[52,53] Recent data have

> **Box 3**
> **Guidelines for shared decision making in the appropriate initiation of and withdrawal from dialysis**
>
> Recommendation #5 from guideline:
>
> "If appropriate, forgo (withhold initiating or withdraw ongoing) dialysis for patients with AKI, CKD, or ESRD in certain, well-defined situations":
>
> - Patients with decision-making capacity, who being fully informed and making voluntary choices, refuse dialysis or request that dialysis be discontinued
> - Patients who no longer possess decision-making capacity who have previously indicated refusal of dialysis in an oral or written advanced directive
> - Patients who no longer possess decision-making capacity and whose properly appointed legal agents/surrogates refuse dialysis or request that it be discontinued
> - Patients with irreversible, profound neurologic impairment such that they lack signs of thought, sensation, purposeful behaviors, and awareness of self and environment
>
> Recommendation #6 from guideline:
>
> "Consider forgoing dialysis for AKI, CKD, or ESRD patients who have a very poor prognosis or for whom dialysis cannot be provided safely":
>
> - Those whose medical condition precludes the technical process of dialysis because the patient is unable to cooperate (eg, advanced dementia patient who pulls out dialysis needles) or because the patient's condition is too unstable (eg, profound hypotension)
> - Those who have a terminal illness from nonrenal causes (acknowledging that some in this condition may perceive benefit from and choose to undergo dialysis)
> - Those with stage 5 CKD older than age 75 years who meet 2 or more of the following statistically significant very poor prognosis criteria: (1) clinicians' response of "No, I would not be surprised" to the surprise question; (2) high comorbidity score; (3) significantly impaired functional status (eg, Karnofsky Performance Status score <40); and (4) severe chronic malnutrition (ie, serum albumin <2.5 g/dL using the bromocresol green method).
>
> *Adapted from* Renal Physician Association shared decision making in the appropriate initiation of and withdrawal from dialysis. 2nd edition. Available at: http://www.renalmd.org/catalogue-item.aspx?id=682. Accessed December 13, 2012.

now demonstrated that older age itself is associated with a greater chance of nonrecovery of renal function back to baseline by the time of hospital discharge, so that survivors are often left with significant CKD.[2,14,60,61]

Few studies have actually quantified the loss of GFR over time after AKI. However, James and colleagues[62] recently demonstrated that the average rate of decline in GFR after mild AKI was 1.0 mL/min per 1.73 m^2 after an episode of moderate AKI, and 2.8 mL/min per 1.73 m^2 after an episode of severe AKI (compared with 0.1 mL/min per 1.73 m^2 in those without AKI). Although this cohort was primarily composed of elderly individuals (mean age 67 in those with AKI), these results among patients undergoing coronary angiography may have limited generalizability to older adults with AKI in the setting of critical illness.

To obtain a sense of the importance of AKI and its lasting effect on renal function, it is worthwhile examining the numbers as they pertain to the sickest cohort of ICU survivors: approximately 1.4 million patients aged 65 years and older are discharged alive after an ICU admission in the United States annually.[63] Because the incidence of AKI in this critically ill population is approximately 30% and the incidence of ESRD after AKI is approximately 26 per 1000 person-years, then approximately 11,000 elderly persons per year are developing new ESRD as a result of AKI in the ICU, representing nearly 11% of total new cases of ESRD annually in the United States.[64] Thus clinicians should be highly vigilant of postdischarge kidney function in the elderly patient after an episode of AKI.

PREVENTION OF AKI IN THE ELDERLY

Given that AKI is a condition associated with significant mortality and morbidity, and that specific therapies are not available to treat AKI after it has occurred, prevention takes on added importance. Prevention of AKI in elderly patients first involves recognizing their increased vulnerability to renal injury, which is associated with the normal age-related decline in GFR (with associated cellular and structural changes in the kidney that occur with aging) or with CKD caused by multiple comorbidities that have accumulated over their life span. A critical aspect in prevention of AKI is to avoid reliance on serum creatinine alone as a measure of renal function and to calculate the estimated GFR using estimating equations (MDRD or CKD-EPI).[65] In this way, patients that may have normal-appearing serum creatinine values are identified with CKD, and their increased risk of AKI can be recognized.

There are some general measures that may ameliorate the risk of AKI in all patients, including minimizing exposure to known nephrotoxins (such as nonsteroidal anti-inflammatory agents, aminoglycosides, or iodinated radiocontrast) and, where possible, monitoring drug levels to ensure that the correct dose is used. Other key measures include maintaining euvolemia and avoiding hypotension, as well as stopping drugs that may alter intrarenal hemodynamics such as angiotensin-converting enzyme inhibitors. Use of the electronic medical record and computer decision support tools, which alert the clinician to the use of potential nephrotoxins and highlight small changes in serum creatinine, may also be of benefit.[66]

For certain potentially nephrotoxic exposures, etiology-specific preventive strategies are available and should be used. Such strategies include:

- Radiocontrast exposure: intravenous hydration with saline or sodium bicarbonate and N-acetylcysteine along with minimization of contrast volume and lower osmolality contrast agents[67]
- Aminoglycoside exposure: once-daily dosing with drug-level monitoring[68]
- Tumor lysis syndrome: intravenous hydration, urinary alkalinization, allopurinol, and rasburicase[69]
- Rhabdomyolysis: intravenous hydration and urinary alkalinization in some cases[70]
- Acyclovir and methotrexate: intravenous hydration[71,72]
- Amphotericin B: use of lipid or liposomal formulations[73]

However, most circumstances that lead to AKI may not be easily preventable. For instance, in one study, in those patients presenting to the emergency department with sepsis the admission serum creatinine was already 2.6 mg/dL, signifying kidney injury before presentation for care.[74,75] In these cases, supportive care will be the major therapeutic focus.

SUMMARY

AKI is an increasing problem for the elderly patient, with dramatic increases in the incidence over the past decade.[5] When AKI does occur, it is associated with both short-term and long-term morbidity and mortality. Although elderly patients tend to have poorer outcomes associated with AKI, most patients can have reasonable outcomes and thus a patient-specific approach to decision making is critical. Wherever possible, preventive strategies should be aggressively pursued and instituted. However, most cases of AKI cannot be easily prevented and in such circumstances, which require dialytic support, recent guidelines for the initiation of dialysis can help frame difficult discussions.

REFERENCES

1. Lamiere N, Van Biesen W, Vanholder R. Acute kidney injury. Lancet 2008;372: 1863–5.
2. Lo LJ, Go AS, Chertow GM, et al. Dialysis-requiring acute renal failure increases the risk of progressive chronic kidney disease. Kidney Int 2009;76:893–9.
3. Hsu CY, Chertow GM, McCulloch CE, et al. Nonrecovery of kidney function and death after acute on chronic renal failure. Clin J Am Soc Nephrol 2009;4:891–8.
4. Liangos O, Wald R, O'Bell JW, et al. Epidemiology and outcomes of acute renal failure in hospitalized patients: a national survey. Clin J Am Soc Nephrol 2006;1: 43–51.
5. Hsu RK, McCulloch CE, Dudley RA, et al. Temporal changes in incidence of dialysis-requiring AKI. J Am Soc Nephrol 2013;24(1):37–42.
6. Feest TJ, Round A, Hamad S. Incidence of severe acute renal failure in adults: results of a community-based study. BMJ 1993;306:481–9.
7. Turney JH, Marshall DH, Brownjohn AM, et al. The evolution of acute renal failure. QJM 1990;74:83–9.
8. Groeneveld AB, Tran DD, Van der Meulen J, et al. Acute renal failure in the intensive care unit: predisposing, complicating factors affecting outcome. Nephron 1991;59:602–7.
9. Pascual J, Orofino L, Liano F, et al. Incidence and prognosis of acute renal failure in older patients. J Am Geriatr Soc 1990;38:25–32.
10. Ali T, Khan I, Simpson W, et al. Incidence and outcome in acute kidney injury: a comprehensive population-based study. J Am Soc Nephrol 2007;18:1292–8.
11. Chronopoulos A, Rosner MH, Cruz DN, et al. Acute kidney injury in elderly intensive care patients: a review. Intensive Care Med 2010;36:1454–64.
12. Uchino S, Kellum JA, Bellomo R, et al. Acute renal failure in critically ill patients: a multinational, multicenter study. JAMA 2005;294:813–8.
13. Bagshaw SM, Laupland KB, Doig CJ, et al. Prognosis for long-term survival and renal recovery in critically ill patients with severe acute renal failure: a population-based study. Crit Care 2005;9:R700–9.
14. Schmitt R, Coca S, Kanbay M, et al. Recovery of kidney function after acute kidney injury in the elderly: a systematic review and meta-analysis. Am J Kidney Dis 2008;52:262–71.
15. Wald R, Quinn RR, Luo J, et al. Chronic dialysis and death among survivors of acute kidney injury requiring dialysis. JAMA 2009;302:1179–85.
16. Macedo E, Bouchard J, Mehta RL. Renal recovery following acute kidney injury. Curr Opin Crit Care 2008;14:660–5.
17. Rosner M. Acute kidney injury in the elderly: pathogenesis, diagnosis and therapy. Aging Health 2009;5:1–10.
18. Turgut F, Balogun RA, Abdel-Rahman EM. Renin-angiotensin-aldosterone system blockade effects on the kidney in the elderly: benefits and limitations. Clin J Am Soc Nephrol 2010;5:1330–9.
19. Coresh J, Selvin E, Stevens LA, et al. Prevalence of chronic kidney disease in the United States. JAMA 2007;298:2038–47.

20. Stevens LA, Li S, Wang C, et al. Prevalence of CKD and comorbid illness in elderly patients in the United States: results from the Kidney Early Evaluation Program (KEEP). Am J Kidney Dis 2010;55:S23–33.

21. Reis AM, Cassiani SH. Adverse drug events in an intensive care unit of a university hospital. Eur J Clin Pharmacol 2011;67:625–32.

22. Goyal VK. Changes with age in the human kidney. Exp Gerontol 1982;17: 321–31.

23. Kaplan C, Pasternack B, Shah H, et al. Age-related incidence of sclerotic glomeruli in human kidneys. Am J Pathol 1975;80:227–34.

24. Lindeman RD, Tobin J, Shock NW. Longitudinal studies on the rate of decline in renal function with age. J Am Geriatr Soc 1985;33:278–85.

25. Epstein M, Hollenberg NK. Age as a determinant of renal sodium conservation in normal man. J Lab Clin Med 1976;87:411–7.

26. Fliser D, Zeier M, Nowack R, et al. Renal functional reserve in healthy elderly subjects. J Am Soc Nephrol 1993;3:1371–7.

27. Baylis C, Fredericks M, Wilson C, et al. Renal vasodilatory response to intravenous glycine in the aging rat kidney. Am J Kidney Dis 1990;15:244–51.

28. Zhang XZ, Qiu C, Baylis C. Sensitivity of the segmental renal arterioles to angiotensin II in the aging rat. Mech Ageing Dev 1997;97:183–92.

29. Reckelhoff JF, Kellum JA, Blanchard EJ, et al. Changes in nitric oxide precursor, l-arginine and metabolites, nitrate and nitrite with aging. Life Sci 1994;55: 1895–901.

30. Miura K, Goldstein RS, Morgan DS, et al. Age-related differences in susceptibilities to renal ischemia in rats. Toxicol Appl Pharmacol 1987;87:284–92.

31. Schmitt R, Marlier A, Cantley LG. Zag expression during aging suppresses proliferation after kidney injury. J Am Soc Nephrol 2008;19:2375–83.

32. Chen G, Bridenbaugh EA, Akintola AD. Increased susceptibility to ischemic injury: identification of candidate genes changed during aging, but corrected by caloric restriction. Am J Physiol Renal Physiol 2007;292:F1272–81.

33. Cheung CM, Ponnusamy A, Anderton JG. Management of acute renal failure in the elderly patient: a clinician's guide. Drugs Aging 2008;25:455–62.

34. Lavizzo-Mourey R, Johnson J, Stolley P. Risk factors for dehydration among elderly nursing home patients. J Am Geriatr Soc 1998;36:213–20.

35. Lamiere N, Verspeelt J, Vanholder R, et al. A review of the pathophysiology, causes and prognosis of acute renal failure in the elderly. Geriatr Nephrol Urol 1991;1:77–87.

36. Perazella MA, Markowitz GS. Drug-induced acute interstitial nephritis. Nat Rev Nephrol 2010;8:461–70.

37. Chang YS. Hypersensitivity reactions to proton pump inhibitors. Curr Opin Allergy Clin Immunol 2012;4:348–53.

38. Preston RA, Stemmer CL, Materson BJ, et al. Renal biopsy in patients 65 years of age or older. Analysis of the results of 334 biopsies. J Am Geriatr Soc 1990; 38:669–78.

39. Rakowski TA, Winchester JF. Renal biopsy in the elderly patient. In: Michelis MF, Preuss HG, editors. Geriatric nephrology. New York: Field Rich; 1986. p. 37–9.

40. Keller F, Michaelis C, Buttner P, et al. Risk factors for long-term survival and renal function in 64 patients with rapidly progressive glomerulonephritis (RPGN). Geriatr Nephrol Urol 1994;4:5–12.

41. Macias-Nunez JF, Lopez-Novoa JM, Martinez-Maldonado M. Acute renal failure in the aged. Semin Nephrol 1996;16:330–6.

42. Pascual J, Liano F. Causes and prognosis of acute renal failure in the very old. Madrid Acute Renal Failure Study Group. J Am Geriatr Soc 1998;46: 721–5.

43. Perazella MA, Parikh CR. How can urine microscopy influence the differential diagnosis of AKI? Clin J Am Soc Nephrol 2009;4:691–3.

44. Perazella MA, Coca SG. Traditional urinary biomarkers in the assessment of hospital-acquired AKI. Clin J Am Soc Nephrol 2012;7:167–74.

45. Dewitte A, Biais M, Petit L, et al. Fractional excretion of urea as a diagnostic index in acute kidney injury in intensive care patients. J Crit Care 2012;27: 505–10.

46. Rosner MH, Bolton WK. Renal function testing. Am J Kidney Dis 2006;47: 174–83.

47. Gill J, Malyuk R, Djurdjev O, et al. Use of GFR equations to adjust drug doses in an elderly multi-ethnic group–a cautionary tale. Nephrol Dial Transplant 2007;22: 2894–9.

48. Singbartl K, Kellum JA. AKI in the ICU: definition, epidemiology, risk stratification and outcomes. Kidney Int 2012;81:819–25.

49. Goldstein SL. Acute kidney injury biomarkers: renal angina and the need for a renal troponin I. BMC Med 2011;9:135.

50. Akposso K, Hertig A, Couprie R, et al. Acute renal failure in patients over 80 years old: 25-years' experience. Intensive Care Med 2000;26:400–6.

51. Van Den Noortgate N, Mouton V, Lamont C, et al. Outcome in a post-cardiac surgery population with acute renal failure requiring dialysis: does age make a difference? Nephrol Dial Transplant 2003;18:732–6.

52. Waikar S, Curhan GC, Wald R, et al. Declining mortality in patients with acute renal failure, 1988 to 2002. J Am Soc Nephrol 2006;17:1143–50.

53. Xue JL, Daniels F, Star RA, et al. Incidence and mortality of acute renal failure in Medicare beneficiaries, 1992 to 2001. J Am Soc Nephrol 2006;17:1135–42.

54. Bagshaw SM, George C, Bellomo R. Changes in the incidence and outcome for early acute kidney injury in a cohort of Australian intensive care units. Crit Care 2007;11:R68.

55. Renal Physician Association shared decision making in the appropriate initiation of and withdrawal from dialysis. 2nd edition. Available at: http://www.renalmd. org/catalogue-item.aspx?id=682. Accessed December 13, 2012.

56. Ricci Z, Cruz D, Ronco C. The RIFLE criteria and mortality in acute kidney injury: a systematic review. Kidney Int 2008;73:538–46.

57. Mehta RL, Pascual MT, Gruta CG, et al. Refining predictive models in critically ill patients with acute renal failure. J Am Soc Nephrol 2002;13:1350–7.

58. Lins RL, Elseviers MM, Daelemans R, et al. Re-evaluation and modification of the Stuivenberg Hospital Acute Renal Failure (SHARF) scoring system for the prognosis of acute renal failure: an independent multicentre, prospective study. Nephrol Dial Transplant 2004;19:2282–8.

59. Chertow GM, Soroko SH, Paganini EP, et al. Mortality after acute renal failure: models for prognostic stratification and risk adjustment. Kidney Int 2006;70: 1120–6.

60. Ishani A, Xue JL, Himmelfarb J, et al. Acute kidney injury increases risk of ESRD among elderly. J Am Soc Nephrol 2009;20:223–8.

61. Newsome BB, Warnock DG, McClellan WM, et al. Long-term risk of mortality and end-stage renal disease among the elderly after small increases in serum creatinine level during hospitalization for acute myocardial infarction. Arch Intern Med 2008;168:609–16.

62. James MT, Ghali WA, Tonelli M, et al. Acute kidney injury following coronary angiography is associated with a long-term decline in kidney function. Kidney Int 2010;78:803–9.
63. Wunsch H, Guerra C, Barnato AE, et al. Three-year outcomes for Medicare beneficiaries who survive intensive care. JAMA 2010;303:849–56.
64. Hsu CY. Where is the epidemic in kidney disease? J Am Soc Nephrol 2010;21: 1607–11.
65. Matsushita K, Mahmoodi BK, Woodward M, et al. Comparison of risk prediction using the CKD-EPI equation and the MDRD study equation for estimated glomerular filtration rate. JAMA 2012;307:1941–51.
66. Chang J, Ronco C, Rosner MH. Computerized decision support systems: improving patient safety in nephrology. Nat Rev Nephrol 2011;7:348–55.
67. Brown JR, Thompson CA. Contrast-induced acute kidney injury: the at-risk patient and protective measures. Curr Cardiol Rep 2010;12:440–5.
68. Pagkalis S, Mantadakis E, Mavros MN, et al. Pharmacological considerations for the proper clinical use of aminoglycosides. Drugs 2011;66:251–9.
69. Howard SC, Jones DP, Pui CH. The tumor lysis syndrome. N Engl J Med 2011; 364:1844–54.
70. Parekh R, Care DA, Tainter CR. Rhabdomyolysis: advances in diagnosis and treatment. Emerg Med Pract 2012;14:1–15.
71. Izzedine H, Launay-Vacher V, Deray G. Antiviral drug-induced nephrotoxicity. Am J Kidney Dis 2005;45:804–17.
72. Perazella MA, Moeckel GW. Nephrotoxicity from chemotherapeutic agents: clinical manifestations, pathobiology and prevention/therapy. Semin Nephrol 2010;30:570–81.
73. Mistro S, Maciel Ide M, de Menezes RG, et al. Does lipid emulsion reduce amphotericin B nephrotoxicity? A systemic review and meta-analysis. Clin Infect Dis 2012;54:1774–7.
74. Rivers E, Nguyen B, Havstad S, et al. Early goal directed therapy in the treatment of sepsis and septic shock. N Engl J Med 2001;345:1368–77.
75. Clinical practice guidelines for acute kidney injury 2012. Available at: http://www.kdigo.org/clinical_practice_guidelines/AKI.php. Accessed December 16, 2012.

An Update on Glomerular Disease in the Elderly

Richard J. Glassock, MD

KEYWORDS

- Glomerulonephritis • Nephrotic syndrome • Immunosuppressive therapy
- Primary glomerular disease • Secondary glomerular disease

KEY POINTS

- Primary and secondary glomerular disease
- Older adult
- Nephrotic syndrome

INTRODUCTION

Both acute and chronic glomerular disease are common causes of disability, hospitalization, and mortality in the elderly population.[1,2] The underlying causes of the glomerular disease in this population are diverse but can be apportioned into those that affect the kidneys primarily (primary glomerular disease) and those in which the kidney damage is a part of a system-wide process (secondary glomerular disease). Regardless of the underlying cause, the clinical features can be condensed into a few clinical syndromes. The comorbid features often associated with advancing age (such as diabetes, atherosclerosis, and congestive heart failure) have important modifying influences on the clinical presentation and course of glomerular disease. This article discusses the common presentations of glomerular disease in the elderly and the clinical features, prognosis, and management of the primary and secondary glomerular diseases in this population of patients.

CLINICAL PRESENTATION

The common clinical syndromes observed at presentation for glomerular disease are shown in **Box 1**.

Acute nephritic syndrome (ANS) is characterized by the abrupt onset of hematuria and proteinuria, often accompanied by edema, hypertension, and reduced renal function (impaired glomerular filtration rate [GFR]). In the elderly, because of concomitant

A version of this article appeared as Glassock, R. Glomerular Disease in the Elderly. Clin Geriatr Med 2009;25(3):413-22.

Department of Medicine, The David Geffen School of Medicine, UCLA, 8 Bethany, Laguna Niguel, Los Angeles, CA 92677, USA

E-mail address: glassock@cox.net

Clin Geriatr Med 29 (2013) 579–591
http://dx.doi.org/10.1016/j.cger.2013.05.007
0749-0690/13/$ – see front matter © 2013 Elsevier Inc. All rights reserved.

> **Box 1**
> **The common clinical syndromes of glomerular disease**
>
> Acute nephritic syndrome
>
> Rapidly progressive glomerulonephritis
>
> Nephrotic syndrome
>
> Asymptomatic hematuria and/or proteinuria
>
> Chronic glomerular disease

chronic ischemic heart disease or preexisting hypertensive cardiomyopathy, marked fluid retention with acute congestive heart failure (pulmonary edema) may be a presenting feature in the ANS, even when the urinary findings are easily overlooked. The disorders evoking the ANS are often accompanied by a tendency for spontaneous recovery, although this is less evident in the elderly compared with younger persons. An antecedent streptococcal (throat or skin) or an active staphylococcal (skin or soft tissue) infection may be documented (poststreptococcal glomerulonephritis or staphylococcal-related glomerulonephritis).

Rapidly progressive glomerulonephritis presents in a more insidious fashion and also manifests hematuria and proteinuria, but is characterized by a progressive and relentless (if untreated) loss of renal function and less evidence of edema and hypertension. Progression to end-stage renal disease (ESRD) may occur in a matter of days or weeks. Although an infection may also be present, such features are usually absent, especially in the elderly. If caused by a systemic disease (such as vasculitis) extrarenal symptoms and signs are commonly present (eg, palpable purpura, lung hemorrhage).

Nephrotic syndrome is characterized by the abrupt or insidious onset of marked proteinuria (usually more than 3.5 g/d up to more than 20 g/d), with or without hematuria, but with a prominent tendency for edema (face and legs), hypoalbuminemia, and hyperlipidemia. Renal function is variable and may be normal or reduced. In the elderly, the peripheral edema may be severe if there is concomitant congestive heart failure or venous insufficiency.

Asymptomatic hematuria and/or proteinuria is characterized by symptom-free (eg, no lower urinary tract symptoms such as dysuria or frequency) excretion of abnormal numbers of intact erythrocytes and/or increased amounts of protein (albumin), or both, in association with normal renal function (adjusted for age), normal blood pressure, and absence of edema. This presentation is often discovered serendipitously during a routine urinalysis, although at times the hematuria may be episodic and gross or macroscopic, thus bringing the patient to the physician's attention. Most often the hematuria is microscopic and persistent or episodic.

Chronic glomerular disease can be said to be present when any of the conditions causing glomerular injury have progressed slowly to definitely impaired renal function (usually a GFR<45 mL/min/1.73 m^2 in the elderly), nearly always with an increased serum creatinine (Scr) concentration. Some degree of proteinuria, often non-nephrotic, and hypertension is also nearly always present.

One feature of the hematuria observed in the glomerular disease syndromes is the excretion of increased numbers of abnormally shaped, smaller than normal (microcytic), poorly hemoglobinized (hypochromic) erythrocytes in the urine.[3] This is also known as dysmorphic or glomerular hematuria. It is a valuable diagnostic tool that requires careful microscopic examination of the urinary sediment (using specials stains or a phase contrast microscope) for accurate detection. When present in larger than normal numbers (>10,000 per mL of uncentrifuged urine or >80% of the erythrocytes in a spun urinary sediment) these dysmorphic erythrocytes are virtually diagnostic of an underlying glomerular disease. Acanthocyturia (erythrocytes with multiple bubble-like projections of the cell membrane) are pathognomonic of glomerulonephritis.

Renal biopsy is often used for definitive diagnosis of the underlying disease process in patients presenting with one or more of the glomerular syndromes. The spectrum of renal diseases encountered in the syndromes enumerated earlier is substantially different in the elderly and the very elderly compared with a younger group of patients.[1,2,4] **Boxes 2** and **3** summarizes the frequency of the more common lesions encountered in the very elderly (more than 80 years of age) when renal biopsies are performed to evaluate clinical renal disease.

PRIMARY GLOMERULAR DISEASE

The lesions that underlie primary glomerular disease are diverse.[4] The relative frequency of the individual glomerular lesions within the spectrum of primary glomerular disease is different in the elderly than in younger patients (see also **Box 2**).[5,6] A stepwise approach to diagnosis of the underlying condition is need, but renal biopsy is often required for definitive diagnosis.[5,6] Five lesions account for more than 80% of the lesions of primary glomerular disease in the elderly: membranous nephropathy (MN); mesangial, endocapillary, or focal proliferative glomerulonephritis (PGN; including immunoglobulin [Ig] A nephropathy); focal and segmental glomerulosclerosis (FSGS); crescentic glomerulonephritis; and minimal change disease (MCD). Membranoproliferative glomerulonephritis (MPGN) is uncommon in the elderly, and is most often found to be caused by a systemic disease (such as a monoclonal gammopathy, autoimmune disease, infections, dysregulation of complement metabolism, or a chronic thrombotic microangiopathy).

Idiopathic MN is the most commonly encountered glomerular lesion in the elderly with primary glomerular disease (it is found in 20%–40% of renal biopsies performed for diagnostic purposes in the presence of nephrotic syndrome in this age group).[1,4,7] Membranous nephropathy is characterized by glomerular capillary wall abnormalities with subepithelial deposits of immune complexes that appear electron dense by ultrastructural analysis. In primary (idiopathic) MN, these deposits are commonly composed of IgG4 antibodies to the muscle-type phospholipase A2 receptor-1 (PLA2R) and the PLA2R antigen located on the podocyte surface.[8]

Box 2
Renal biopsy diagnosis in the very elderly (more than 80 years of age)

Pauci-immune crescentic glomerulonephritis: 18%

Focal and segmental glomerulosclerosis plus hypertensive nephrosclerosis: 7%

Hypertensive nephrosclerosis: 7%

Immunoglobulin (Ig) A nephropathy: 7%

Membranous nephropathy: 7%

Amyloidosis: 6%

Minimal change disease: 4%

Myeloma cast nephropathy: 4%

Data from Moutzouris DA, Herlitz L, Appel GA, et al. Renal biopsy in the very elderly. Clin J Am Soc Nephrol 2009;4:1073–82.

> **Box 3**
> **The frequency of primary glomerular lesions in the older adult (according to renal biopsy series)**
>
> Membranous nephropathy: 28%
>
> Mesangial proliferative glomerulonephritis[a]: 24%
>
> Crescentic glomerulonephritis (pauci-immune): 13%
>
> Minimal change disease: 10%
>
> Focal and segmental glomerulosclerosis: 9%
>
> Membranoproliferative glomerulonephritis: 8%
>
> Endocapillary (acute) proliferative glomerulonephritis: 4%
>
> Chronic glomerulonephritis (not otherwise specified): 4%
>
> [a] Including IgA nephropathy and pure mesangial proliferative glomerulonephritis.
> *Data from* Faubert PF, Porush JG. Primary glomerular disease. In: Faubert PF, Porush JG, editors. Renal disease in the elderly. 2nd edition. New York: Marcel Dekker; 1998. p. 129–73.

Most patients with MN present with typical features of the nephrotic syndrome (>85%), but a few present with asymptomatic proteinuria, often without hematuria. Persistence of proteinuria is the rule, but spontaneous remissions occur in 20% to 30% of patients, depending in part on the magnitude of initial proteinuria.[9] Continuing nephrotic-range proteinuria, particularly more than about 4 g/d, can be associated with a slowly progressive course to ESRD over many years. A greater magnitude of proteinuria and longer persistence is strongly associated with a greater risk of eventual ESRD.[10] Concomitant hyperlipidemia may aggravate an underlying tendency to progressive atherosclerosis and cardiovascular disease. There is also a marked tendency to thromboembolic diseases, including deep venous thrombosis of the legs, and renal vein thrombosis, sometimes with nonfatal or fatal pulmonary embolism.[11]

The diagnosis of the primary (idiopathic) forms of MN is aided by the detection of autoantibodies to PLA2R1 in the circulation. Such autoantibodies are found in 70% to 80% of patients with idiopathic MN.[12]

Conservative management (salt restriction; loop-acting diuretics; antihypertensive agents, mainly angiotensin-converting enzyme inhibitors [ACEi], angiotensin receptor blockers [ARB], or direct renin inhibitors [DRI]) is indicated when proteinuria is modest (<4 g/d), the symptoms of nephrotic syndrome are tolerable and manageable, or features suggesting progressive disease (declining GFR) are absent. Concomitant therapy with a statin to help reduce the hypercholesterolemia is often indicated. Prophylactic anticoagulants may be indicated when the serum albumin level is low (<2.8 g/dL), if the patient has had a prior thromboembolic event, or has another thrombophilic disorder and is at low risk of a bleeding complication of anticoagulation.[13] Patients with marked proteinuria (>4 g/d for 6 months or longer), those with severe symptomatic nephrotic syndrome, or those with progressive renal disease (Scr levels of 1.5–2.5 mg/dL) are candidates for specific therapy.[14] Several choices are available for initial therapy and the selection of one or the other for initial treatment depends on individual preferences and the importance of side effects. Two regimens are commonly considered. Cyclical oral cyclophosphamide (or chlorambucil, with cyclophosphamide as the preferred agent) and glucocorticoids for 6 months (the Ponticelli regimen) are preferred for initial therapy.[14] This regimen has a high success rate (complete or partial remissions in more than 80%) and delays the onset of progressive renal failure. However, in the elderly it may be associated with a higher risk of leucopenia and viral infections (eg, herpes zoster). Concomitant increase of Scr increases this risk and lower doses of cyclophosphamide (50%–75% of the usual recommended dose) are used in the regimen. Relapses occur in about 20% to 30% of patients after initial success. This regimen may be repeated for severe relapses, but no more than once. As an alternative, treatment may be initiated with a calcineurin inhibitor (CNI; cyclosporine or tacrolimus), alone as monotherapy or combined with low-dose steroids for 4 to 6 months, providing that the initial renal function is normal or near normal. The success rate for initial remission using a CNI is equivalent to that of the Ponticelli regimen, but relapses are higher (around 60%–70%) when the therapy is tapered or discontinued and therefore treatment must be prolonged to maintain remission, exposing the patient to the potential nephrotoxicity of these agents. Many patients become CNI dependent, with relapses developing when the CNI is reduced to less than a critical threshold of efficacy. Tacrolimus may produce more stable remissions and seems to be effective even without concomitant steroids. Other alternative agents, not yet fully evaluated for long-term benefits and risks, include synthetic or natural adrenocorticotropic hormone gel (twice weekly for 6 months to 1 year); intravenous courses of rituximab (a monoclonal anti-CD20 B-cell antibody), and mycophenolate mofetil (MMF) plus steroids.[13,15–18] Failure to respond to the Ponticelli regimen or to a CNI is a common indication for these second-line therapies, but the response is difficult to predict. Resistance to treatment with one class of agent does not reliably predict resistance to another class of agent. Concomitant use of rituximab and a CNI (in CNI-dependent patients) has produced long-term remission free of relapse, but this has not yet been evaluated in a suitable randomized clinical trial.[19] A lasting complete or partial remission resulting from any treatment regimen is associated with marked protection from ESRD. Recurrences of MN in renal transplants can develop in 15% to 20% of cases, but few elderly patients are candidates for such a procedure.

Mesangial, endocapillary, or focal proliferative glomerulonephritis is most commonly a manifestation of an underlying streptococcal, staphylococcal, or viral infection.[20] Poststreptococcal glomerulonephritis is not a benign disease in the elderly. It may provoke a fatal bout of acute congestive heart failure. Treatment is primarily supportive with diuretics, bed rest, and salt restriction. Staphylococcal-related glomerulonephritis may be associated with IgA deposits in the glomeruli and has a poor prognosis, especially in the concomltant presence of diabetes.

IgA nephropathy is common in the elderly (accounting for about 15% of diagnoses of primary glomerular disease).[5,21] Its prognosis and treatment in the elderly are largely unknown, but persistence of proteinuria greater than 500 mg/d and more severe glomerular and/or tubulointerstitial lesion in renal biopsy is associated with a tendency for progression to ESRD. Too few elderly patients have been included in randomized trials to help to guide treatment decisions. The standard therapy for IgA nephropathy is maximum dosage of an ACEi/ARB or DRI. Combination of an ACEi and an ARB or a DRI may be more effective in lowering protein excretion over the short term, but the long-term benefits and risk of such combination therapy are unknown and side effects may be increased in the elderly with underlying cardiovascular disease. Patients with proteinuria persisting at more than 1.0 g/d after 6 months of optimal angiotensin II inhibition therapy and Scr less than 1.5 mg/dL could be treated with cyclical oral and intravenous prednisone (Pozzi regimen).[21] Patients with progressive disease could also be treated with low-dose sequential cyclophosphamide-azathioprine and glucocorticoids (Ballardie-Roberts regimen),[21] but the safety and efficacy of this approach in the elderly is largely unknown. Fish oils (purified omega-3 fatty acids) also have beneficial effects, but this has not been consistently shown in clinical trials. Such treatment is generally well tolerated, with few side effects other than gastrointestinal upset (eructations) and an unpleasant odor of the skin. Azathioprine is ineffective and MMF has only been successful in Asian patients. The effects of rituximab are largely unknown. Beneficial effects of CNI have been reported but randomized clinical trials are lacking.[22] IgA nephropathy frequently recurs in the renal allograft but this does not have a major effect on graft or patient survival, except when severe disease (eg, crescentic glomerulonephritis) is present.[23]

FSGS is a common lesion found to underlie proteinuria and the nephrotic syndrome in the geriatric population.[1,5,24] The primary form of the lesion is characterized by a segmental sclerosis affecting some but not all glomeruli. IgM and C3 deposits are commonly seen in the sclerosed segments by immunofluorescence microscopy, and ultrastructural analysis shows diffuse effacement of the foot processes. It may be difficult to clearly separate this lesion from MCD on pathologic grounds alone, because of the common superimposition of global glomerulosclerosis and vascular lesions in the elderly kidney. Patients with the FSGS lesion tend to have an insidious onset of nephrotic syndrome, often present with some degree of renal impairment, and frequently have hypertension. This lesion tends to be uncommon in the very elderly (>80 years of age).[4,5] Proteinuria may be marked (as much as 20 g/d) and progressive renal failure is common if marked proteinuria persists. Patients with non-nephrotic proteinuria (<about 2 g/d) largely have a benign evolution and can be managed conservatively with diuretics and ACEi, ARB, or DRI. Management is problematic for those with persistent nephrotic-range proteinuria because there are few randomized controlled trials that include elderly patients to help in decision making. A prolonged course of oral glucocorticoids (4–6 months) is often used, but side effects are frequent and often disabling, especially in the elderly (osteoporosis, diabetes, sleep disturbances, easy bruising, myalgias, fatigue). About 30% to 60% of patients enter a complete or partial remission with such treatment, but relapses are common when treatment is withdrawn.[23] Because of poor tolerability of prolonged steroid treatment, some prefer to initiate therapy with a combination of a CNI (cyclosporine or tacrolimus) and low-dose alternate-day oral steroids (along with concomitant maximum-dose ACEi, ARB, or DRI). This regimen can be complicated by further impairment of renal function and dosage of CNI frequently needs to be adjusted. About 40% to 60% of steroid-resistant patients treated with a CNI regimen experience a remission (mostly partial) and relapses are common. Alkylating agents (cyclophosphamide or chlorambucil) are of no value in steroid-resistant FSGS and should be avoided. Oral MMF, given with steroids (such as high-dose dexamethasone), has been beneficial, similar to CNI, the long-term benefits are unknown.[25] Combinations of MMF and a CNI have been used on an anecdotal basis with good results, but publication bias is a concern. Rituximab has shown some limited benefit, but no controlled trails are yet available. Patients who are refractory to all treatment measures generally progress to ESRD over 2 to 4 years. The subvariant of FSGS known as collapsing glomerulopathy has a poorer prognosis and tends to be less responsive to treatment when glomerular involvement is severe (>25% of glomeruli involved with collapsing lesions).[26] The disease may recur in the transplanted kidney in up to 40% of cases, but this is seldom an issue in the elderly.

Crescentic glomerulonephritis is one of the more common primary glomerular lesions found in elderly subjects (40%–50% of all lesions in some series).[1,5] This lesion is characterized by abundant proliferation of the cells lining the Bowman space and glomerular podocytes (forming crescents) and by necrotizing lesions in the glomerular capillaries. Three distinct pathogenetic mechanisms are operative: (1) antiglomerular basement membrane (GBM) antibodies producing a linear deposit of IgG along the capillary walls; (2) immune complex deposits producing a granular pattern of immuno-globulin along the capillary walls and mesangium, and (3) pauci-immune lesions with relative absence of immunoglobulin in glomeruli.[27] Pauci-immune lesions are frequently (>80%) associated with circulating antineutrophil cytoplasmic autoanti-bodies (ANCA) directed to myeloperoxidase or proteinase 3 in the azurophilic granules of leukocytes. The linear deposit of IgG is commonly caused by anti-GBM autoanti-body production, whereas the immune complex lesions are commonly caused by lupus nephritis, IgA nephropathy, or infections. These lesions are frequently associ-ated with the clinical syndrome of rapidly progressive glomerulonephritis. The diag-nosis of crescentic glomerulonephritis should always be suspected when hematuria and proteinuria are found and the Scr is increasing rapidly. Urgent specific diagnosis of the type of glomerulonephritis by serology (anti-GBM and ANCA in particular) and/ or renal biopsy is indicated. The pauci-immune form is the commonest type (>75% of crescentic glomerulonephritis observed in the older and elderly subject), but infre-quently anti-GBM or immune complex types can be encountered.

In the absence of early and aggressive therapy, most patients either die or develop irreversible ESRD. Renal biopsies showing few normal glomeruli or advanced glomer-ulosclerosis and interstitial fibrosis suggest an adverse prognosis for eventual recov-ery. Treatment needs to be initiated early for maximal benefit. For the pauci-immune lesion, remission induction therapy consists of oral or intravenous glucocorticoids, oral or intravenous cyclophosphamide, and in some cases intensive plasma exchange (if patients have an acute and severe loss of GFR or are dialysis dependent for <2 weeks). About 60% of patients treated with this regimen experience a complete or partial remission within 3 to 6 months. If the initial Scr is less than 4.0 mg/dL, treat-ment with intravenous rituximab can achieve equivalent results.[28] After induction of remission with cyclophosphamide and steroids or rituximab, the intensity of treatment may be diminished and maintenance of remission with oral azathioprine (or MMF) and low-dose glucocorticoids in those initially treated with cyclophosphamide and ste-roids may be sufficient. No chemical maintenance therapy may be required for those treated initially with rituximab, but repeated courses of rituximab (every 4–6 months) may be required to prevent relapses. Relapses are common, particularly in the variety associated with antibodies to proteinase 3. The overall response rate to this therapy following these induction regimens is more than 60% (and as high as 80%), but complications are frequent and the mortality remains high (more than 20%). The elderly are especially vulnerable to infectious complications. If the burden of real or potential side effects is judged to be excessive, it is better to withhold therapy and plan for dialysis. The lesions of crescentic glomerulonephritis caused by anti-GBM or ANCA can uncommonly recur in the renal allograft.

MCD in many ways is the most difficult lesion to identify with certainty as a cause for the nephrotic syndrome in the elderly.[1,2,4,5,29] In younger persons, the lesions are mainly seen at the level of the electron microscope, at which diffuse foot process effacement is evident. Light microscopy is normal or shows only mild mesangial changes and immunofluorescence microscopy is negative or reveals only wisps of IgM in the mesangium. In the elderly, superimposed lesions of arteriolonephroscle-rosis and global glomerulosclerosis may result in imprecision when rendering diagnosis of MCD (by light microscopy alone). MCD is a common cause of the idiopathic nephrotic syndrome in the older adult, accounting for about 10% to 20% of all cases, diminishing in frequency with even more advancing age. MCD in the older adult is typi-cally associated with the abrupt onset of a full-blown nephrotic syndrome with scant hematuria and normal blood pressure for the person's age. A characteristic feature of

MCD in the elderly is its common association with (mostly reversible) acute kidney failure injury (AKI).[30] Episodes of AKI develop in about one-third of cases, often abruptly at the onset of disease. The AKI is commonly spontaneously reversible, but permanent renal failure has also been observed. The reasons underlying this propensity for AKI with MCD in older adults are not well understood. Except for this tendency, MCD in the older individual is similar to that found in younger subjects in terms of presentation and course. However, spontaneous remissions of the nephrotic syndrome seem to be uncommon in the elderly.

The treatment of MCD in the older adult is not well known, again because of a paucity of randomized controlled trials in the aged. However, if the nephrotic syndrome is severe, treatment with oral glucocorticoids, given once daily or every other day in doses of 1 mg/kg/d (maximum dose of 80 mg daily or 120 mg every other day) are usually given. Treatment must be prolonged in many cases, for 16 to 20 weeks, to achieve a remission. With this treatment regimen, about 75% of older patients can be expected to enter a remission. However, relapses may develop as treatment is withdrawn, although infrequently in the elderly compared with younger persons. Adjunctive use of short-term oral cyclophosphamide (1.5–2.0 mg/kg/d for 8–10 weeks) or a CNI-based regimen (similar to that used in FSGS) can be offered for those few patients with frequent recurrences, but there are side effects and potential risks.[29] Resistance to the effects of steroids usually indicates an underlying lesion of FSGS, missed in the original renal biopsy. Overall the prognosis for maintenance of good renal function is good for MCD in the elderly, except if AKI supervenes. Deep venous thrombosis and thromboembolism may occur during episodes of full-blown nephrotic syndrome.

SECONDARY GLOMERULAR DISEASE

The secondary glomerular diseases that affect the elderly are diverse (**Box 4**).[1,2] These entities can produce any or all of the clinical syndromes previously enumerated. Often the character of the systemic (extrarenal) features give clues to the correct diagnosis, but in many cases these clues are nonspecific and of little diagnostic help. Because renal biopsies are only done for diagnosis when the causes of the clinical syndrome are not immediately self-evident, the frequency of secondary lesions among collected renal biopsy series gives a distorted view of their true prevalence. For example, diabetic glomerulosclerosis (DGS; discussed elsewhere in this issue), both diffuse and nodular, caused by type 2 diabetes mellitus, is among the most common causes of

---

Box 4
Common secondary glomerular diseases in the elderly

Diabetic glomerulosclerosis (diffuse and nodular types) type 2 diabetes

Systemic necrotizing and crescentic glomerulonephritis (antineutrophil cytoplasmic autoantibody positive)

Systemic amyloidosis (AL type, primary and secondary to multiple myeloma)

Nonamyloid monoclonal immunoglobulin deposition diseases (light chain, heavy chain, light-heavy chain, cryoglobulinemia)

Idiopathic (nondiabetic) nodular glomerulosclerosis

Malignancy-related glomerulopathy (MN, focal and segmental glomerulosclerosis, MCD)

Drug-related glomerular disease (nonsteroidal antiinflammatory agents, cancer chemotherapeutic agents, bisphosphonates [Pamidronate], interferons)

glomerulopathy in the elderly, but is less common (usually about 5%–10%) in renal biopsy series. In addition, DGS may also be associated with (superimposed on) other primary or secondary glomerular diseases. The most important causes of secondary glomerular disease that are more common in the elderly than in younger subjects are amyloidosis, nonamyloid monoclonal immunoglobulin deposition diseases, nondiabetic (idiopathic) nodular glomerulosclerosis, Goodpasture disease (anti-GBM antibody nephritis), and systemic necrotizing polyangiitis. Lupus nephritis is uncommon in the elderly. Membranous nephropathy and, to a lesser extent, FSGS and MCD, may also develop as a consequence of malignancies in older individuals.[31,32] About 25% of patients with MN diagnosed when older than 65 years have an underlying malignancy, most often a carcinoma (breast, stomach, lung, or colon).[31,32] Hodgkin disease, thymomas, lymphomas, and other solid malignancies or leukemias may be associated with MCD or FSGS. Drugs such as nonsteroidal antiinflammatory agents, consumed more commonly by the elderly for a variety of symptoms, can also evoke glomerular disease (MCD and MN). Therapeutic agents, used in the treatment of cancer and its complications in the elderly, such as interferon or bisphosphonates (pamidronate), can also induce glomerular lesions (MCD and collapsing FSGS). Viral infections such as human immunodeficiency virus, hepatitis B, and hepatitis C cause glomerular lesions (MN and MPGN), but are more common in younger than in older subjects. However, chronic hepatitis C infection is a common cause of mixed IgG/IgM cryoglobulinemia in elderly patients (often complicated by a vasculitis), particularly in women.[33]

Amyloidosis is a cause of the nephrotic syndrome in about 10% to 15% of elderly patients.[34] It may present as a renal disease (nephrotic syndrome most commonly) without any extrarenal manifestations but more frequently some clues to the correct diagnosis are present, such as carpal tunnel syndrome, macroglossia, easy bruising, postural hypotension, diarrhea, organomegaly, cardiac disease, or liver disease. In the elderly, AL amyloidosis is the most common disease, but rarely AA amyloidosis or even hereditary amyloidosis (especially fibrinogen alpha chain mutations) may be the cause. The Congo red stain is positive and 10-nm to 12-nm nonbranching fibrils are found on electron microscopy. Marked proteinuria (up to 20 g/d or more) and some impairment of renal function with mild hypertension is the rule. Plasma levels of free monoclonal immunoglobulin light chains (typically lambda) are frequently increased (>80%) and a monoclonal paraprotein can often be found in the urine (most often lambda light chains). About 10% of patients with AL amyloidosis have a frank multiple myeloma on bone marrow examination or bone survey. Nephrotic syndrome and reduced renal function are ominous prognostic signs and, in the absence of therapy, nearly all patients die or progress to ESRD in a matter of a few years from discovery. Although the elderly have a high risk of serious side effects and complications, an attempt at therapy is usually warranted. Such attempts include high-dose melphalan plus steroids, or bortezomib and lenalidomide (a congener of thalidomide). Autologous bone marrow (or peripheral stem cell) transplantation is poorly tolerated in the elderly, especially if cardiac involvement is present, and this approach (although curative) may be too risky to be applied to the elderly population with renal AL amyloidosis.

Nonamyloid monoclonal immunoglobulin deposition diseases (MIDD) are also a common cause of renal disease in the older population.[35] They may collectively account for 10% to 15% of cases. The diseases consist of light chain MIDD (usually kappa light chain), heavy chain MIDD, light-heavy chain MIDD, IgG MIDD, monoclonal cryoglobulinemia, crystal cryoglobulinemia, and immunotactoid glomerulopathy. These diseases share in common the deposition of a nonamyloid monoclonal protein (Congo red stain negative) in the glomerular capillaries, lacking the β pleated sheet conformation, causing structural and functional deficits including nephrotic syndrome and progressive renal failure. Identification of the relevant monoclonal protein by immunochemical means is essential for the correct diagnosis, and chemotherapy is needed to reduce the production of the abnormal protein from a neoplastic clone of B cells and/or plasma cells. Laser capture microscopy and mass spectroscopy are increasingly valuable tools to identify the nature of the deposits in this group of diseases.[36]

Idiopathic (nondiabetic) nodular glomerulosclerosis is a recently described condition in which the pathologic findings of nodular DGS are found in patients who have no evidence of diabetes mellitus.[37] The patients tend to be elderly women with a strong history of smoking and hypertension. The pathogenesis is unknown and the prognosis is poor. No effective treatment is available, other than control of blood pressure and stopping smoking.

Goodpasture disease (anti-GBM nephritis) is an uncommon disorder characterized by crescentic glomerulonephritis (discussed earlier) and circulating antibodies to GBM, often accompanied by diffuse alveolar hemorrhage.[38] In the elderly it is chiefly found in women and overt (alveolar hemorrhage can be observed in less than 50% of cases). There may be a coexisting ANCA-associated nephritis/vasculitis in as many as 20% of cases.[39] With extensive crescents, the prognosis for recovery is poor without aggressive therapy. Treatment consists of oral cyclophosphamide (in reduced dosage), oral and intravenous glucocorticoids, and aggressive plasma exchange (14 sessions for several weeks). Circulating antibody levels decrease quickly but renal recovery depends on the extent of damage at the time treatment is begun. Maintenance immunosuppressive therapy is usually not required unless concomitant ANCA-associated disease is present. Dialysis-dependent patients with Scr greater than 6 mg/dL have only a 10% chance or less of recovery of renal function.[40] Life-threatening pulmonary hemorrhage is best treated by high-dose steroids and intensive plasma exchange, which may be life saving.

Systemic pauci-immune necrotizing and crescentic polyangiitis is among the most common secondary glomerular diseases affecting the elderly.[1,2,4,5] This condition is similar to the renal-limited form (discussed earlier). The systemic forms are (1) granulomatous polyangiitis (GPA; formerly called Wegener granulomatosus) affecting the kidneys, lungs, upper airways, sinuses, sclera, and auditory canal with evident granulomas in the affected vascular tissue; and (2) microscopic polyangiitis (MPA), also affecting the kidneys, lungs, skin, and joints, but without vascular tissue granulomas. Both are strongly associated (>90%) with ANCA; mostly antiproteinase 3 in GPA and antimyeloperoxidase in MPA. Systemic features of fever, cough, myalgias, pulmonary hemorrhage, necrotizing cutaneous angiitis, sinusitis, and upper and lower airway disease can be present. The treatment is identical to that described earlier for renal-limited necrotizing and crescentic glomerulonephritis but the prognosis may be poorer because of the multiorgan involvement. Patients who are dialysis dependent for less than 2 weeks are likely to benefit from the addition of intensive plasma exchange but the risk of complications is great, especially in the infirm. Courses of rituximab are emerging as an alternative to cyclophosphamide-glucocorticoid regimens, especially in relapsing disease.[27] CNI or MMF may, rarely, be useful, but only anecdotes are available to guide decisions in this area.

SUMMARY

This brief recapitulation of the major features of glomerular disease in the geriatric population provides several lessons. The importance of careful examination of the urinary sediment for dysmorphic erythrocytes as a diagnostic tool in glomerular disease needs to be emphasized. A high degree of suspicion for underlying glomerular disease needs to be present when hematuria and proteinuria are present concomitantly and an increasing serum creatinine should be viewed with a sense of urgency. The atypical clinical features of acute and chronic glomerular disease in the elderly should be remembered. The common causes of nephrotic syndrome, such as MN, FSGS, MCD, and amyloidosis need to be remembered in patients with edema and marked proteinuria. The unusual predilection of the elderly to develop rapidly progressive glomerulonephritis caused by both renal-limited and systemic forms of necrotizing and crescentic glomerulonephritis (often antineutrophil cytoplasmic autoantibody positive) needs to be appreciated. The development of glomerular disease caused by an underlying neoplastic process, such as monoclonal immunoglobulin deposition disease or a carcinoma, also needs to be remembered. In addition, many clinical trials have failed to include sufficient numbers of elderly persons, which makes it difficult to translate therapeutic recommendations from the young to the old. The risks of aggressive treatment of glomerular disease may also be enhanced in older persons and this needs to be recognized in therapeutic decision making. However, many effective and reasonably safe treatment regimens are available to ameliorate the adverse consequences of acute, progressive, and chronic glomerular disease in the geriatric population. They must be used with care and with full recognition of their potential benefits and hazards in this uniquely vulnerable population.

REFERENCES

1. Faubert PF, Porush JG. Primary glomerular disease. In: Faubert PF, Porush JG, editors. Renal disease in the elderly. 2nd edition. New York: Marcel Dekker, Inc; 1998. p. 129–73.
2. Glassock RJ. Glomerular disease in the elderly population. In: Oreopoulos DG, Hazzard WR, Luke R, editors. Nephrology and geriatrics integrated. Dordrecht (The Netherlands): Kluwer Academic Publishers; 2000. p. 57–66.
3. Becker GJ, Fairley KF. Urinalysis. In: Massry S, Glassock R, editors. Textbook of nephrology. 4th edition. Philadelphia: Lippincott Williams and Wilkins; 2001. p. 1765–83.
4. Yokoyama H, Sugiyama H, Sato H, et al, Committee for the Standardization of Renal Pathological Diagnosis and for Renal Biopsy and Disease Registry of the Japanese Society of Nephrology, and the Progressive Renal Disease Research of the Ministry of Health, Labour and Welfare of Japan. Renal disease in the elderly and the very elderly Japanese: analysis of the Japan Renal Biopsy Registry (J-RBR). Clin Exp Nephrol 2012;16(6):903–20.
5. Ponticelli C, Glassock RJ. Treatment of primary glomerulonephritis. 2nd edition. Oxford (United Kingdom): Oxford University Press; 2009. p. 1–476.
6. Moutzouris DA, Herlitz L, Appel GA, et al. Renal biopsy in the very elderly. Clin J Am Soc Nephrol 2009;4:1073–82.
7. Vendemia F. The diagnosis of renal disease in elderly patients. What role is there for renal biopsy? In: Nunez JF, Cameron JS, Oreopoulos DG, editors. The aging kidney in health and disease. New York: Springer; 2008. p. 307–28.
8. Beck LH Jr, Salant DJ. Membranous nephropathy: recent travels and new roads ahead. Kidney Int 2010;77(9):765–70.
9. Polanco N, Gutiérrez E, Covarsí A, et al, Grupo de Estudio de las Enfermedades Glomerulares de la Sociedad Española de Nefrología. Spontaneous remission of nephrotic syndrome in idiopathic membranous nephropathy. J Am Soc Nephrol 2010;21(4):697–704.

10. Pei Y, Cattran D, Greenwood C. Predicting chronic renal insufficiency in idiopathic membranous glomerulonephritis. Kidney Int 1992;42:960–6.
11. Lionaki S, Derebail VK, Hogan SL, et al. Venous thromboembolism in patients with membranous nephropathy. Clin J Am Soc Nephrol 2012;7(1):43–51.
12. Qin W, Beck LH Jr, Zeng C, et al. Anti-phospholipase A2 receptor antibody in membranous nephropathy. J Am Soc Nephrol 2011;22(6):1137–43.
13. Glassock RJ. Prophylactic anti-coagulation in nephrotic syndrome: a clinical conundrum. J Am Soc Nephrol 2007;18:2221–5.
14. Passerini P, Ponticelli C. Membranous nephropathy. In: Ponticelli C, Glassock R, editors. Treatment of primary glomerular disease. 2nd edition. Oxford (United Kingdom): Oxford University Press; 2009. p. 261–312.
15. Bomback AS, Canetta PA, Beck LH Jr, et al. Treatment of resistant glomerular diseases with adrenocorticotropic hormone gel: a prospective trial. Am J Nephrol 2012;36(1):58–67.
16. Ruggenenti P, Cravedi P, Chianca A, et al. Rituximab in idiopathic membranous nephropathy. J Am Soc Nephrol 2012;23(8):1416–25.
17. Chan TM, Lin AW, Tang SC, et al. Prospective controlled study on mycophenolate mofetil and prednisolone in the treatment of membranous nephropathy with nephrotic syndrome. Nephrology (Carlton) 2007;12(6):576–81.
18. Dussol B, Morange S, Burtey S, et al. Mycophenolate mofetil monotherapy in membranous nephropathy: a 1-year randomized controlled trial. Am J Kidney Dis 2008;52(4):699–705.
19. Segarra A, Praga M, Ramos N, et al. Successful treatment of membranous glomerulonephritis with rituximab in calcineurin inhibitor-dependent patients. Clin J Am Soc Nephrol 2009;4:1083–8.
20. Moroni G, Ponticelli C. Acute post-infectious glomerulonephritis. In: Ponticelli C, Glassock R, editors. Treatment of primary glomerular disease. 2nd edition. Oxford (United Kingdom): Oxford University Press; 2009. p. 153–78.
21. Glassock RJ, Lee G. Immunoglobulin A nephropathy. In: Ponticelli C, Glassock R, editors. Treatment of primary glomerular disease. 2nd edition. Oxford (United Kingdom): Oxford University Press; 2009. p. 313–74.
22. Shin JI, Lim BJ, Kim PK, et al. Effects of cyclosporin A therapy combined with steroids and angiotensin converting enzyme inhibitors on childhood IgA nephropathy. J Korean Med Sci 2010;25(5):723–7.
23. Ponticelli C, Glassock RJ. Posttransplant recurrence of primary glomerulonephritis. Clin J Am Soc Nephrol 2010;5(12):2363–72.
24. Scolari F, Ponticelli C. Focal and segmental glomerulosclerosis. In: Ponticelli C, Glassock R, editors. Treatment of primary glomerular disease. 2nd edition. Oxford (United Kingdom): Oxford University Press; 2009. p. 215–60.
25. Gipson DS, Trachtman H, Kaskel FJ, et al. Clinical trial of focal segmental glomerulosclerosis in children and young adults. Kidney Int 2011;80(8):868–78.
26. Klemmer PJ, Chalermskulrat W, Reif MS, et al. Plasmapheresis therapy for diffuse alveolar hemorrhage in patients with small-vessel vasculitis. Am J Kidney Dis 2003;42(6):1149–53.
27. Nachman P, Glassock R. Crescentic glomerulonephritis. In: Ponticelli C, Glassock R, editors. Treatment of primary glomerular disease. 2nd edition. Oxford (United Kingdom): Oxford University press; 2009. p. 399–434.
28. Stone JH, Merkel PA, Spiera R, et al, RAVE-ITN Research Group. Rituximab versus cyclophosphamide for ANCA-associated vasculitis. N Engl J Med 2010; 363(3):221–32.

29. Coppo R, Ponticelli C. Minimal change nephropathy. In: Ponticelli C, Glassock R, editors. Treatment of primary glomerular disease. 2nd edition. Oxford (United Kingdom): Oxford University Press; 2009. p. 179–214.

30. Brandão Tavares M, da Chagas de Almeida M, Martins RT, et al. Acute tubular necrosis and renal failure in patients with glomerular disease. Ren Fail 2012; 34(10):1252–7.

31. Beck LH Jr. Membranous nephropathy and malignancy. Semin Nephrol 2010; 30(6):635–44.

32. Bjoneklett R, Vikse BE, Svarstad E, et al. Long-term risk of cancer in membranous nephropathy patients. Am J Kidney Dis 2007;50:396–403.

33. Terrier B, Cacoub P. Cryoglobulinemia vasculitis: an update. Curr Opin Rheumatol 2013;25(1):10–8.

34. Dember LM. Amyloidosis-associated kidney disease. J Am Soc Nephrol 2006;17: 3458–71.

35. Lin J, Markowitz GA, Valeri AM, et al. Renal immunoglobulin deposition disease: the clinical spectrum. J Am Soc Nephrol 2001;12:1482–92.

36. Sethi S, Theis JD, Vrana JA, et al. Laser microdissection and proteomic analysis of amyloidosis, cryoglobulinemic GN, fibrillary GN, and immunotactoid glomerulopathy. Clin J Am Soc Nephrol 2013. [Epub ahead of print].

37. Nasr SH, D'Agati VD. Nodular glomerulosclerosis in the nondiabetic smoker. J Am Soc Nephrol 2007;18:2032–6.

38. Cui Z, Zhao MH. Advances in human antiglomerular basement membrane disease. Nat Rev Nephrol 2011;7(12):697–705.

39. Levy JB, Hammad T, Coulthart A, et al. Clinical features and outcome of patients with both ANCA and anti-GBM antibodies. Kidney Int 2004;66(4):1535–40.

40. Levy JB, Turner AN, Rees AJ, et al. Long-term outcome of anti-glomerular basement membrane antibody disease treated with plasma exchange and immunosuppression. Ann Intern Med 2001;134(11):1033–42.

Hypertension in the Elderly
Unique Challenges and Management

Faruk Turgut, MD[a], Yusuf Yesil, MD[b], Rasheed A. Balogun, MD[c],
Emaad M. Abdel-Rahman, MD, PhD[c],*

KEYWORDS

- Hypertension • Elderly • Pathophysiology • Epidemiology • Management

KEY POINTS

- Although many aspects of hypertension diagnosis and treatment are similar in younger and older patients, there are many relevant issues that are unique to the elderly and require attention while treating the elderly.
- Most recommendations in managing elderly hypertensive patients are based on expert opinion because of limited evidence available.
- Key considerations in the management of hypertension in the elderly include selection of a target blood pressure and selection of agents used to attain the chosen target.
- Elderly patients with hypertension and diabetes may be treated with either angiotensin-converting enzyme inhibitors (ACEIs), angiotensin-receptor blockers (ARBs), calcium channel blockers, thiazide diuretics, and elderly patients with hypertension and chronic kidney disease should be treated with ACEIs or ARBs, with close follow-up of kidney function and potassium level.

INTRODUCTION

Blood pressure (BP) is strongly and directly associated with cardiovascular morbidity and mortality from young adulthood to older age groups.[1] With the increased life expectancy over the last few decades, elderly individuals, defined as aged 65 years and older, are the fastest increasing cohort in the worldwide population.[2] The attendant increase in prevalence of hypertension and other comorbidities is a major concern as the population ages.

Lowering high BP is beneficial and untreated or poorly controlled hypertension is associated with permanent morbidity and mortality. Lowering high BP not only improves survival but also reduces incidence of strokes and other cardiovascular

[a] Department of Nephrology, School of Medicine, Mustafa Kemal University, 31034, Hatay, Turkey; [b] Division of Geriatric Medicine, Department of Internal Medicine, School of Medicine, Hacettepe University, 06100, Ankara, Turkey; [c] Division of Nephrology, University of Virginia, Box 800133, Charlottesville, VA 22908, USA
* Corresponding author.
E-mail address: ea6n@virginia.edu

Clin Geriatr Med 29 (2013) 593–609
http://dx.doi.org/10.1016/j.cger.2013.05.002
0749-0690/13/$ – see front matter © 2013 Elsevier Inc. All rights reserved.

events, including heart failure even in very elderly patient population groups.[3–5] Antihypertensive therapy, when indicated, is an important intervention to minimize functional decline and disability in the elderly.

Many aspects of hypertension diagnosis and treatment are similar in younger and older patients; however, there are many relevant issues that require attention while treating the elderly. This situation is mainly because of differences in physiology and concurrent medical conditions, which pose additional medical challenges when managing elderly patients with hypertension. It seems that, generally, older hypertensive patients are more likely to be aware of their diagnosis of hypertension and more likely to be treated; however, once treated, they are less likely to achieve good BP control, compared with younger hypertensive patients.[6] The lower rate of BP control shows that hypertension in the elderly is still a significant problem that deserves more attention. Although it is well established that both systolic and diastolic hypertension must be treated in the elderly,[5,7,8] the preferred agents to use have not necessarily been clearly identified, which may also contribute to lower rates of hypertension control in this patient population. On the other hand, the high prevalence of both cardiovascular and noncardiovascular comorbidity among the elderly dictates the need for greater vigilance to avoid treatment-related adverse effects, including electrolyte disturbances and renal dysfunction. This review highlights the diagnosis and management of hypertension in the elderly, including current relevant information and concepts.

EPIDEMIOLOGY

Arterial hypertension is highly prevalent in the elderly. BP continues to increase with advancing age, and data from the Framingham Heart Study, in men and women free of hypertension at 55 years of age, indicate that the remaining lifetime risks for development of hypertension to 80 years are 93% and 91%, respectively.[9] According to the Seventh Report of the Joint National Committee on Prevention, Detection, Evaluation and Treatment of High Blood Pressure (JNC-7), hypertension occurs in more than two-thirds of elderly individuals.[7] It has also been shown that 60% of all adults aged 60 to 69 years and up to 77% of those older than 80 years have hypertension.[10] Hypertension prevalence is higher in women than in men older than 65 years (**Table 1**). The severity of hypertension increases markedly with advancing age in women as well.[11]

PATHOPHYSIOLOGY

Age-related BP increases are mainly attributable to changes in arterial structure and function that accompany aging (**Fig. 1**).[12] These changes include increase in vessel wall collagen content and collagen fiber cross-linking, loss of vascular smooth muscle cells, calcium deposition, disruption, and thinning of the elastic fibers.[13] Impaired

Table 1		
Epidemiology of hypertension in the elderly		
Hypertension in Elderly	**Source (Ref.)**	**Epidemiology (%)**
Risk for developing hypertension in elderly	Framingham study[9]	Males: 93 Females: 91
Prevalence of hypertension in elderly	JNC-7[7] Otschega et al,[10] 2007	>66 Age 60–69 y: 60 Age >80 y: 77

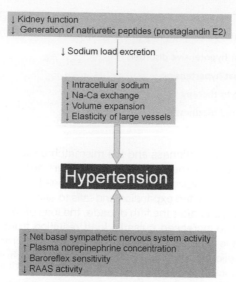

↓ Kidney function
↓ Generation of natriuretic peptides (prostaglandin E2)

↓ Sodium load excretion

↑ Intracellular sodium
↓ Na-Ca exchange
↑ Volume expansion
↓ Elasticity of large vessels

Hypertension

↑ Net basal sympathetic nervous system activity
↑ Plasma norepinephrine concentration
↓ Baroreflex sensitivity
↓ RAAS activity

Fig. 1. Changes in arterial structure and function that accompany aging.

vasodilatation caused by endothelial dysfunction also contributes to the arterial stiffness that is common in elderly hypertensive patients.[14]

Another potential mechanism that may contribute to the development of hypertension in the elderly is increased salt sensitivity. As a result of an aging-related decline in renal function as well as increased dietary sodium load, BP increases (see **Fig. 1**).[15,16] Decrease in activity of membrane sodium, potassium, and calcium adenosine triphosphate pumps in older adults leads to an excess of intracellular calcium and sustained vasoconstriction, thereby increasing vascular resistance.[17,18] Decreased activity of the sodium pump and polymorphisms of the angiotensin-converting enzyme (ACE) gene also play a role in the pathogenesis of salt sensitivity in the elderly.[19–25] A decrease of estrogen levels after menopause enhances salt sensitivity in elderly women.[26,27]

Neurohormonal mechanisms do not play a major role in BP regulation in older adults compared with younger individuals. However, with aging, there is a progressive decline in baseline plasma renin activity and renin secretion after stimuli such as standing, salt depletion, or furosemide administration.[28–31] In addition, sympathetic nervous system activity increases with advancing age and peripheral plasma norepinephrine concentration is higher than in younger individuals. All of these mechanisms a play key role in the pathogenesis of hypertension in the elderly.

White Coat Hypertension

White coat hypertension is defined as persistently increased BP in the doctor's office (≥140/90 mm Hg) in a patient with a normal daytime ambulatory BP (≤135/85 mm Hg).[7] White coat hypertension is common in the elderly, and ambulatory BP monitoring should be considered to avoid overtreatment in suspected hypertensive patients (**Box 1**).[32]

Isolated Systolic Hypertension

Isolated systolic hypertension is defined as the presence of systolic BP of greater than or equal to 160 mm Hg with a diastolic BP less than 90 mm Hg.[33] Isolated systolic hypertension accounts for 60% to 80% of cases of hypertension in the elderly.[34,35]

Box 1
Indications for ambulatory BP monitoring in the elderly

Suspicion of syncope or hypotensive disorders

Evaluation of white coat hypertension

Evaluation of response to therapy

Evaluation of vertigo and dizziness

As a result, increased aortic stiffness and the mismatch between aortic diameter and blood flow contribute to the expanding of pulse pressure and development of systolic hypertension. As a result of aging, systolic BP increases linearly because of an aged arterial tree, which shows limited expansion and fails to effectively buffer the pressures generated by the heart, and after the fifth decade, the loss of recoil during diastole reduces diastolic BP. The increased pulsatile load resulting from the increased pulse pressure, damages the heart and the vasculature, thus, increasing cardiovascular risk.[8,16] Isolated systolic hypertension is associated with a 2-fold to 4-fold increase in the risk of cardiovascular morbidity and mortality.[36,37]

Brachial versus central BP

Increased arterial stiffness is one of the main determinants of isolated systolic hypertension. Because atherosclerosis, a marker for cardiovascular events, may be the cause of arterial stiffening, central BP may be a better indicator of cardiovascular events in the elderly. Pini and colleagues[38] followed 864 community-dwelling elderly individuals for 8 years. Clinical assessment including echocardiography, carotid ultrasonography, applanation tonometry, and cardiovascular events were obtained. These investigators showed that higher carotid systolic BP but not brachial pressures independently predicted cardiovascular mortality. Similarly, higher carotid systolic BP and pulse pressure predicted cardiovascular events, whereas brachial pressure failed to predict cardiovascular events. These results suggest a superior prognostic importance of carotid BP over brachial BP.

Pseudohypertension

Pseudohypertension is a falsely increased systolic BP caused by atherosclerotic and other vascular changes associated with age. Pseudohypertension should be suspected in elderly patients with long-standing refractory hypertension and still with no organ damage. Confirmation of pseudohypertension may require direct measurement of intra-arterial BP.

Masked hypertension

Masked hypertension is defined as increased ambulatory or home BP despite a normal office BP.[39] Masked hypertension is an emerging clinical entity predisposing to subclinical organ damage and to increased cardiovascular risk.[40,41] The prevalence of masked hypertension is difficult to determine precisely, but seems to lie between 10% and 41% in the elderly.[40–42] This particular form of hypertension may be underdiagnosed in the elderly during their routine medical examination. Therefore, widespread use of home BP monitoring should be encouraged in the elderly population.

THERAPEUTIC CHALLENGES IN THE ELDERLY

The major goals of lowering BP in elderly patients include reduction of mortality and cardiovascular events and slowing progression of chronic kidney disease (CKD).

Suboptimal or outright therapy failure is common in the elderly, often because of real or perceived side effects and increased pill burden, resulting in poor adherence, which is a major issue in antihypertensive therapy. Nonadherence often results in failing to reach BP targets and affects outcomes in the elderly.

The elderly population is more likely to take nonsteroidal antiinflammatory drugs, which are known to increase BP by inhibiting the production of vasodilatory prostaglandins.[43] Therefore, BP control may be difficult in those patients using nonsteroidal antiinflammatory drugs, and usage should be minimized in this patient group. Other drugs that can make BP control more difficult should also be checked in this population (**Table 2**).

Lowering BP too much is associated with more side effects and may be dangerous in the elderly. It may impair mental function, leading to confusion and sleepiness, and may cause additional morbidity, such as ischemic optic neuropathy. Orthostatic hypotension may be aggravated by the aggressive therapy.

Orthostatic Hypotension

Orthostatic hypotension and postprandial hypotension are also limiting factors to the use of antihypertensive drugs in the elderly. Orthostatic hypotension, a significant independent predictor of mortality, is more common in the elderly and its prevalence is found to be as high as 20% of elderly patients.[44] Elderly patients, particularly those who are frail, may be more likely to experience injury as a result of an episode of hypotension. Falls in the elderly from dizziness, and so forth, can be fatal, so more attention needs to be paid to the medication and doses. It is especially important to monitor those patients taking α-blockers, as many elderly men with prostatism do, or a high-dose diuretic, because these 2 classes of drugs are more likely to cause postural hypotension.

Most of the trials showing benefit from the treatment of hypertension in the elderly were performed in relatively fit patients. Greater caution should be applied to frail patients, and treatment may be withheld if orthostatic hypotension is limiting.

BP TARGETS IN THE ELDERLY

The American College of Cardiology Foundation(ACCF)/American Heart Association (AHA) 2011 expert consensus, for the first time, stratified the elderly into young old

Table 2	
Medications used by elderly patients that can increase BP	
Nonsteroidal antiinflammatory drugs	Acetylsalicylic acid Ibuprofen Naproxen
Steroids	Prednisone Methylprednisolone Dexamethasone
Antidepressants	Venlafaxine Bupropion Desipramine
Cough and cold medications (decongestants)	Pseudoephedrine Phenylephrine
Migraine medications	Ergotamine Zolmitriptan Sumatriptan

(65–74 years), older old (75–84 years), and old old (≥85 years).[8] In the light of this recommendation, age-specific target BPs may be described. The ACCF/AHA stated that the BP should be reduced to less than 140/90 mm Hg in all elderly patients with uncomplicated hypertension based on expert opinion.[8] Nevertheless, for those who cannot tolerate this level and those old old population, a systolic BP of 140 to 150 mm Hg, if tolerated, is acceptable from data from HYVET (the Hypertension in the Very Elderly Trial).[3,8] Systolic BP lower than 130 mm Hg should be avoided in the elderly 80 years of age or older.[8] Too low a diastolic BP may decrease coronary perfusion and possibly increase cardiovascular risk.[45] In the SHEP (The Systolic Hypertension in the Elderly Program) trial, elderly patients with lower diastolic BP have higher cardiovascular events.[37]

The general recommended BP goal in complicated hypertension is less than 130/80 mm Hg in the general population. Whether the elderly patients with certain comorbidities (such as CKD, diabetes, heart failure) benefit from more stringent target BPs has been tested in some trials. In the ACCORD BP (Action to Control Cardiovascular Risk in Diabetes Blood Pressure) trial, intensive antihypertensive therapy (BP <120 mm Hg vs 140 mm Hg), particularly in hypertensive diabetic patients, was found to be associated with more serious side effects than standard therapy and may even be more deleterious in elderly patients.[46] Similarly, systolic BP less than 115 mm Hg and diastolic BP less then 65 mm Hg was found in the INVEST (International Verapamil SR/Trandolapril) study[47] to be associated with increased mortality in predominantly elderly hypertensive patients with coronary artery disease .

A target BP less than 130/80 mm Hg is recommended for elderly hypertensive patients with CKD based on expert opinion and observational data.[8] Most elderly patients with CKD have isolated systolic hypertension. Thus, theoretically, treatment of their systolic hypertension may have the unintended effect of lowering diastolic pressure to suboptimal levels, leading to impaired perfusion during diastole. Furthermore, it is not clear that slowing progression of CKD is always the most meaningful goal of antihypertensive therapy in older patients with a low estimated glomerular filtration rate, because their risk for other outcomes such as cardiovascular events, disability, and cognitive insufficiency is often higher than that for end-stage renal disease. None of the trials used to support the safety of BP targets lower than usual in patients with CKD enrolled any participants older than 70 years. Thus, the safety of treating to a BP level lower than usual in elderly patients is not known.

In deciding whether to target a BP lower than usual in older patients, the clinician must consider each individual patient's likelihood of experiencing progressive loss of renal function and mortality in relation to their age peers and in the context of their risk for other health outcomes and their risk for adverse events as a result of BP decrease.

NONPHARMACOLOGIC THERAPY

Treatment of hypertension generally begins with nonpharmacologic therapy, which continues to be an important component in hypertension management. All guidelines recommend lifestyle modifications for elderly patients whose BP exceeds prescribed thresholds and who are at moderate or high cardiovascular disease risk. Lifestyle changes should include weight reduction (results in a 5–mm Hg to 20–mm Hg decrease in systolic BP per 10 kg less), increased physical activity (4–mm Hg to 9–mm Hg decrease in systolic BP), smoking cessation, and sodium and alcohol restriction.[7,48,49] Lifestyle changes may be enough to control for milder forms of hypertension and may even reduce the doses of antihypertensive drugs.[8] Elderly patients are relatively more salt sensitive because of their reduced ability to excrete a sodium load. TONE (Trial of Non-pharmacologic Interventions in the Elderly) showed that the combination of weight loss and sodium restriction decreased both systolic (5.3 ± 1.2 mm Hg) and diastolic BP (3.4 ± 0.8 mm Hg) in obese, elderly hypertensive patients.[50] BP-lowering effects of dietary sodium restriction are generally greater in older than young adults.[8] When lifestyle measures fail to decrease BP to goal, pharmacologic therapy should be initiated.

PHARMACOLOGIC THERAPY

Pharmacologic therapy should generally be started if the systolic BP is persistently 140 mm Hg or greater or the diastolic BP is persistently 90 mm Hg or greater in the office and at home, despite attempted nonpharmacologic therapy. When BP is greater than 20/10 mm Hg higher than goal, it should be started with 2 antihypertensive drugs.[8] According to the ACCF/AHA, the initial antihypertensive drug should be started at the lowest dose and gradually be increased depending on the BP response up to the maximum tolerated dose.[8] After reaching full dose, if BP is still uncontrolled, a second drug from another class should be added. In the National Institute for Health and Care Excellence (NICE) guidelines, antihypertensive therapy is recommended for those at any age who have stage 2 hypertension, but starting antihypertensive therapy is recommended only for patients younger than 80 years with stage 1 hypertension if they have target organ damage or diabetes renal disease or established cardiovascular disease.[51]

Several prospective studies attested to the safety and efficacy of antihypertensive drugs in reducing mortality and morbidity in the elderly. An overview of selected outcome trials in the elderly is shown in **Table 3**.

CHOICE OF ANTIHYPERTENSIVE AGENTS IN THE ELDERLY

In the management of hypertension, the choice of specific antihypertensive drug depends on efficacy, tolerability, presence of specific comorbidities, and cost. In general, 3 classes of drugs are considered as first-line therapy for the treatment of uncomplicated hypertension in the elderly.

1. Diuretics (low-dose thiazide diuretics)
2. Long-acting calcium channel blockers (CCBs) (especially dihydropyridines)
3. ACE inhibitors (ACEIs) or angiotensin-receptor blockers (ARBs)

Most elderly patients require 2 or more antihypertensive drugs. If orthostatic or postprandial hypotension develops, the dose of antihypertensive drug may need to be reduced or another antihypertensive drug should be used. Assessment of subclinical organ damage during treatment is crucial, because the goal is to protect patients from progressing organ damage and potentially from cardiovascular events. The choice of therapy for elderly patients with complicated hypertension differs from uncomplicated hypertension (**Table 4**). Treatment decisions should be guided by the presence of compelling indications, and drug combinations may be needed in complicated hypertension.

DIURETICS

Diuretics control hypertension by inhibiting reabsorption of sodium and chloride ions from the tubules in the kidney. Diuretics decrease BP by decreasing intravascular volume and peripheral vascular resistance. Thiazides are the preferred diuretics, from data showing their efficacy in reducing stroke and cardiovascular mortality in

Table 3
Selected clinical studies that have evaluated the effects of antihypertensive therapy in the elderly

Studies	N	Age Range (Mean Age, y)	Drugs	Mean Follow-Up	Results
ANBP 2 (The Australian National Blood Pressure study)	6083	65–84 (72)	ACEI vs diuretics	4.1 y	↓ CV events ↔ Stroke ↓ CV mortality
HYVET	3845	80–105 (84)	Indapamide + perindopril	1.8 y	↓ CV events (34%) ↓ Stroke (46%) ↓ CV mortality (27%)
MRC (Medical Research Council Trial)	4396	65–74 (70)	Atenolol vs HCTZ or amiloride	5.8 y	↓ CV events (%) ↓ Stroke (%) ↓ CV mortality (%)
SHEP	4736	≥60 (72)	Chlortalidone	>5 y	↓ CV events (32%) ↓ Stroke (36%) ↔ CV mortality
STOP-HTN (The Swedish Trial in Old Patients with Hypertension study)	1627	70–84 (76)	Atenolol + HCTZ or amiloride or metoprolol or pindolol	25 mo	↓ CV events (40%) ↓ Stroke (46%) ↓ CV mortality (43%)
Syst-China (Systolic Hypertension in China study)	2394	≥60 (67)	Nitrendipine ± captopril or HCTZ	3 y	↓ CV events ↓ Stroke ↔ CV mortality
Syst-Eur (The Systolic Hypertension in Europe study)	4695	≥60 (70)	Nitrendipine ± enalapril or HCTZ	24 mo	↓ CV events (26%) ↓ Stroke (42%) ↓ CV mortality (23%)
SCOPE (The Study on Cognition and Prognosis in the Elderly)	4937	70–89 (76)	Candesartan	44.6 mo	↓ CV events (11%) ↓ Stroke (24%) ↔ CV mortality
JATOS (the Japanese Trial to Assess Optimal Systolic Blood Pressure in Elderly Hypertensive Patients)	4418	65–85 (75)	Efonidipine hydrochloride	2 y	↔ CV mortality
VALISH (The Valsartan in Elderly Isolated Systolic Hypertension study)	3079	70–84 (76)	Valsartan	2.85 y	↔ CV mortality

Abbreviations: ↓, reduction in outcome; ↔, no difference in outcome; ACEI, angiotensin-converting enzyme inhibitor; ARB, angiotensin-II receptor blocker; HCTZ, hydrochlorothiazide.

elderly patients with hypertension.[52] A recent retrospective study by Dhalla and colleagues compared the relative safety and effectiveness of 2 thiazide diuretics (chlorthalidone and hydrochlorothiazide) used in the management of elderly. The primary outcome was a composite of mortality and hospitalization for cardiovascular events. Safety outcomes included electrolyte problems (hyponatremia and hypokalemia) as well as hospitalization.[53] No statistical difference was observed in the primary outcome between the 2 drugs. Chlorthalidone in older adults was associated with a

Table 4
The choice of therapy for elderly patients with complicated hypertension

Complicated Disease	First Choice	Second Choice	Third Choice
CAD (stable angina or previous MI)	β-Blocker	Long-acting dihydropyridine CCB	ACEI (if LV dysfunction)
Systolic HF	Diuretic, ACEI (ARB, if ACEI not tolerated)	β-Blocker	Aldosterone antagonist
Asymptomatic LV systolic dysfunction	ACEI and β-blocker		
LV hypertrophy	ACEI, ARB		
Stroke or TIA	ACEI and diuretic		
Aortic aneurysm	ACEI or ARB and β-blocker		
Diabetes and nephropathy	ACEI or ARB		

Abbreviations: CAD, coronary artery disease; HF, heart failure; LV, left ventricular; MI, myocardial infarction; TIA, transient ischemic attack.

greater incidence of electrolyte abnormalities compared with hydrochlorothiazide. Until there is a prospective randomized trial comparing these 2 drugs, it is reasonable to use either drug to achieve adequate BP control, carefully watching the electrolyte when using either drugs and more so when using chlorthalidone.

Prospective studies also showed that diuretics reduced cardiovascular morbidity and mortality in elderly diabetic hypertensive patients.[54,55] The landmark study that proved that isolated systolic hypertension should be treated was SHEP.[52] In this trial, patients with systolic BP levels 160 mm Hg and greater and diastolic BP levels less than 90 mm Hg, documented over several visits, were randomly assigned to anti-hypertensive therapy with a thiazide-type diuretic (chlorthalidone) or placebo. In the active arm, atenolol or reserpine was added to attain the desired BP (143/68 mm Hg). Almost one-half of the patients reached the target BP solely with low-dose chlorthalidone. The study showed greater reductions in BP in the treated group. Furthermore, the incidence of stroke was significantly lower in the treatment group (5.5% vs 8.2%) as well as the incidence of cardiac events, although it was not statistically significant in all age groups, including those patients aged 80 years and older. There were few adverse effects of active treatment. Only about 4% of patients had hypokalemia (as defined by a potassium level <3.2 mEq/L). Again, a meta-analysis of 10 trials with β-blockers and diuretics in patients aged 60 years or older[56] showed that diuretic therapy was superior to β-blockade with regard to all end points, suggesting that β-blockers should not be considered as first-line therapy.

Diuretics are generally well tolerated; however, they can cause various metabolic side effects, including electrolyte abnormalities (hypokalemia, hyponatremia), dyslipidemia, insulin resistance, and new-onset diabetes mellitus.[57] However, no significant increase was found in any outcome (stroke, coronary artery disease, heart failure, end-stage renal disease, total mortality) in patients using diuretic therapy who developed new-onset diabetes mellitus.[58] Diuretics are not recommended in patients with baseline electrolyte abnormalities, and serum sodium and potassium levels should be monitored. The ACCF/AHA recommends that initial therapy should, if possible, be a diuretic and if another class is prescribed as a first-line therapy, the second drug should always be a diuretic.[8]

CCBS

CCBs are widely used as antihypertensive agents because of their efficacy, metabolic neutrality, and good side effect profile. Recent prospective randomized studies attested to the safety of CCBs in the elderly. In the Syst-Eur (Systolic Hypertension in Europe) study,[33] elderly patients with isolated systolic hypertension were randomized to the dihydropyridine CCB nitrendipine or placebo. The study was stopped earlier than anticipated because of a significant reduction in stroke. In the ACCOMPLISH (Avoiding Cardiovascular Events through Combination Therapy in Patients Living with Systolic Hypertension) study, a combination of ACEI and CCB was shown to be superior (relative risk reduction of 21% for cardiovascular events) to ACEI plus diuretic combination independent of age (either >80 years or <80 years).[59]

In general, CCBs seem well tolerated by the elderly. CCBs dilate coronary and peripheral arteries. Thus, most adverse effects relate to consequences of vasodilation, including ankle edema, headache, and postural hypotension. Moreover, nondihydropyridines can precipitate heart blocks in the elderly, with underlying conduction defects.

CCBs were recommended as initial therapy in the NICE guidelines for all patients older than 55 years. If a CCB is not suitable because of side effect (edema or intolerance), or if there is evidence of heart failure or a high risk of heart failure, thiazidelike diuretic is recommended.[51]

RENIN-ANGIOTENSIN-ALDOSTERONE SYSTEM BLOCKERS

The renin-angiotensin-aldosterone system (RAAS) is a major regulatory system of both cardiovascular and renal functions. Overactivity of the RAAS is associated with the development of hypertension, cardiovascular events, and CKD.[60–62] Based on a large body of evidence, inhibition of the RAAS is a commonly used method to decrease BP and to reduce the incidence of end-organ damage. Several studies have reported that the blockade of the RAAS by ACEIs, ARBs, and direct renin inhibitors (DRI) showed beneficial effects on hypertension, CKD, and cardiovascular disease in patients with CKD, including the elderly.[63–67] Thus, this group of drugs is widely included in clinical guidelines to manage hypertension and other cardiovascular diseases.[7,8,68,69] In applying these guidelines to the management of elderly patients with hypertension, ACEIs and ARBs may be used in elderly population.[66]

ACEIs and ARBs should be considered first-line or combination therapy for elderly hypertensive patients with diabetes or nephropathy.[8] In a subgroup analysis among participants older than 65 years enrolled in the Reduction of Endpoints in Non-insulin dependent diabetes mellitus with the Angiotensin II Antagonist Losartan (RENAAL) trial, a trial among type II diabetics with macroalbuminuria, losartan was similarly renoprotective in these older participants as it was in the overall study population, suggesting that this agent is equally efficacious in elderly patients with albuminuria.[70] HYVET investigated the effects of antihypertensive treatment on stroke, mortality, and other outcomes in very elderly hypertensive patients (age ≥80 years).[3] A total of 3845 patients have been randomized to placebo or active treatment, starting with indapamide 1.5 mg sustained release and adding the ACEI perindopril if required. HYVET was stopped prematurely because of encouraging preliminary results observed in the active treatment group. The results of the HYVET study showed that antihypertensive therapy with indapamide with or without perindopril reduces the risks of death from stroke and death from any cause in very elderly patients. However, patients recruited were generally healthier than those in general population and target BP was 150/80 mm Hg in this study. Therefore, benefits from lower targets still need to be established.

The DRI aliskiren is highly specific for rennin, and it inhibits catalytic activity of renin by binding to its active site. The safety and tolerability of aliskiren were studied in elderly patients with systolic hypertension.[67] Aliskiren has been shown to be not only effective but also well tolerated in elderly hypertensive patients. However, there is no evidence to justify replacing an ACEI or ARB with aliskiren for renal outcomes in elderly patients.

Prescription of RAAS blockers in elderly patients mandates careful monitoring for side effects, including acute renal failure and hyperkalemia, often requiring extra laboratory testing and clinic visits after initiation of these agents and after any change in dose. In addition, administration of these agents in elderly patients with CKD may require dietary modification and chronic administration of ion-exchange resins and can also limit the use of other medications that also increase serum potassium (eg, spironolactone). Potentially dangerous potassium disturbances complicated by the consequences of a noncontrolled diet, concomitant drugs, and other associated chronic disease are more common among elderly patients with impaired renal function. Consequently, safety issues regarding use of these drugs particularly in patients with CKD require more caution in the elderly population. It is well documented that patients with CKD in whom treatment with ACEIs or ARBs is indicated should be checked for serum creatinine and potassium levels 7 to 10 days after prescription.

The effect of blockade of RAAS in elderly patients seems to be effective. In deciding whether to treat an older patient with CKD with an ACEI or ARB to slow progression of CKD, the clinician should consider whether the patient has proteinuria, whether their CKD is clearly progressive, whether they have other health concerns or priorities that might make another antihypertensive agent preferable, and whether the additional burden that these agents may impose is justified and acceptable to the patient.

Combination of RAAS Blockers in the Elderly

Compliance rates decrease as the number of drugs increases. Thus, combination therapy improves compliance as well as efficacy. There are no clinical studies that show superiority of 1 combination compared with the other. With the limited available data, unless there is compelling indication, combination of RAAS blockers should be avoided in the elderly. A diuretic, β-blocker, ACEIs (or ARBs), and aldosterone antagonist may be combined (in the absence of hyperkalemia or significant renal dysfunction) in elderly hypertensive patients with systolic heart failure.[8] There are no outcome studies that show a benefit on survival, or progression of CKD, in elderly patients who are treated with ACEIs or ARBs in combination with aldosterone antagonists.

As aging occurs, angiotensin levels decrease. With a diuretic therapy, the low renin status changes to a higher renin level. Thus, when combination therapies are needed, ACEI or ARB combination with a diuretic is effective.[7] Conversely, Bakris and colleagues[71] argued that initial antihypertensive treatment with combination of ACEI and CCB should be considered in preference to ACEI and diuretic combination based on the ACCOMPLISH trial results. In this study, 11,506 hypertensive elderly patients (defined as >60 years, with mean age 68 years) from 5 countries were randomized into 2 treatment arms: ACEI + CCB (amlodipine) versus ACEI + diuretic (hydrochlorothiazide). Patients were followed for 36 months. The trial was terminated early because of superior efficacy of the ACEI + CCB combination over the ACEI + diuretic combination. A major criticism of the study was the exclusion of patients with heart failure, with probable worse heart failure outcomes with amlodipine as shown in ALLHAT (Antihypertensive and Lipid-Lowering Treatment to Prevent Heart Attack Trial). Another concern was that the ACEI + CCB arm achieved a greater blood pressure reduction, raising the question whether the better BP control, rather than the specific drug was the reason for the better outcome noted in patients treated with the ACE + amlodipine combination.

β-BLOCKERS

β-blockers are not recommended as first-line treatment of hypertension. They may have a role in combination therapy, particularly in elderly patients with complicated hypertension.[72] The class of β-blockers is heterogeneous, and all the drugs in the class may be not be the same. Metoprolol, carvedilol, and nebivolol may differ from other β-blockers in terms of efficacy and side effects.[73] The initial choice may be a β-blocker in elderly hypertensive patients with coronary artery disease (stable angina or previous myocardial infarction).[8] Despite their BP-lowering effect, β-blockers failed to reduce strokes and cardiac events in the elderly.[56] Current evidence does not suggest considering β-blockers for primary therapy for hypertension in the absence of a specific indication (eg, heart failure or myocardial infarction) in the elderly.[8]

OTHER ANTIHYPERTENSIVE DRUGS

α-Blockers (doxasosin), centrally acting drugs (clonidine, reserpine), and nonspecific vasodilators (hydralazine, minoxidil) should not be used as first-line antihypertensive therapy in the elderly because of their possible adverse effects.[8,74] In terms of adverse effects, α-blockers are not as bad as central α-agonists like clonidine, and adverse effects seem to be decreased if an α-blocker is combined with a β-blocker. α-Blockers are generally used for prostate hypertrophy and caution should be paid to avoid orthostatic hypotension.

SUMMARY

Because of limited evidence available in managing elderly hypertensive patients, most recommendations are based on expert opinion. Key considerations in the management of hypertension include selection of a target BP and selection of agents used to attain the chosen target. Elderly patients with hypertension and diabetes may be treated with ACEIs, ARBs, CCBs, thiazide diuretics. Elderly patients with hypertension and CKD should be treated with ACEIs or ARBs.

In addition to treating hypertension, the physician must treat other modifiable cardiovascular risk factors in patients with or without diabetes mellitus or CKD to reduce cardiovascular events and mortality. According to the negative effects of hypertension on the quality of life among the elderly, diagnostic and treatment centers for hypertension prevention and management need to be established, the prevalence of hypertension in different groups should be determined based on age, sex, location, and level of education, and the medical staff have to be educated about the importance, complications, and new therapeutic strategies to treat hypertension.

REFERENCES

1. Lewington S, Clarke R, Qizilbash N, et al. Age-specific relevance of usual blood pressure to vascular mortality: a meta-analysis of individual data for one million adults in 61 prospective studies. Lancet 2002;360(9349):1903–13.

2. Available at: www.census.gov/compendia/statab/2010/tables/10s0034.pdf. Accessed January 2013.
3. Beckett NS, Peters R, Fletcher AE, et al. Treatment of hypertension in patients 80 years of age or older. N Engl J Med 2008;358(18):1887–98.
4. Kostis JB, Davis BR, Cutler J, et al. Prevention of heart failure by antihypertensive drug treatment in older persons with isolated systolic hypertension. SHEP Cooperative Research Group. JAMA 1997;278(3):212–6.
5. Staessen JA, Wang JG, Thijs L. Cardiovascular protection and blood pressure reduction: a meta-analysis. Lancet 2001;358(9290):1305–15.
6. Egan BM, Zhao Y, Axon RN. US trends in prevalence, awareness, treatment, and control of hypertension, 1988-2008. JAMA 2010;303(20):2043–50.
7. Chobanian AV, Bakris GL, Black HR, et al. The Seventh Report of the Joint National Committee on Prevention, Detection, Evaluation, and Treatment of High Blood Pressure: the JNC 7 report. JAMA 2003;289(19):2560–72.
8. Aronow WS, Fleg JL, Pepine CJ, et al. ACCF/AHA 2011 expert consensus document on hypertension in the elderly: a report of the American College of Cardiology Foundation Task Force on clinical expert consensus documents developed in collaboration with the American Academy of Neurology, American Geriatrics Society, American Society for Preventive Cardiology, American Society of Hypertension, American Society of Nephrology, Association of Black Cardiologists, and European Society of Hypertension. J Am Coll Cardiol 2011; 57(20):2037–114.
9. Vasan RS, Beiser A, Seshadri S, et al. Residual lifetime risk for developing hypertension in middle-aged women and men: the Framingham Heart Study. JAMA 2002;287(8):1003–10.
10. Ostchega Y, Dillon CF, Hughes JP, et al. Trends in hypertension prevalence, awareness, treatment, and control in older U.S. adults: data from the National Health and Nutrition Examination Survey 1988 to 2004. J Am Geriatr Soc 2007;55(7):1056–65.
11. Ong KL, Tso AW, Lam KS, et al. Gender difference in blood pressure control and cardiovascular risk factors in Americans with diagnosed hypertension. Hypertension 2008;51(4):1142–8.
12. O'Rourke MF, Hashimoto J. Mechanical factors in arterial aging: a clinical perspective. J Am Coll Cardiol 2007;50(1):1–13.
13. Dao HH, Essalihi R, Bouvet C, et al. Evolution and modulation of age-related medial elastocalcinosis: impact on large artery stiffness and isolated systolic hypertension. Cardiovasc Res 2005;66(2):307–17.
14. Wallace SM, Yasmin, McEniery CM, et al. Isolated systolic hypertension is characterized by increased aortic stiffness and endothelial dysfunction. Hypertension 2007;50(1):228–33.
15. Epstein M, Hollenberg NK. Age as a determinant of renal sodium conservation in normal man. J Lab Clin Med 1976;87(3):411–7.
16. Acelajado MC, Oparil S. Hypertension in the elderly. Clin Geriatr Med 2009; 25(3):391–412.
17. Volkov VS, Romanova NP, Poseliugina OB. Salt consumption and arterial hypertension. Kardiologiia 2003;43(11):36–7 [in Russian].
18. Zemel MB, Sowers JR. Salt sensitivity and systemic hypertension in the elderly. Am J Cardiol 1988;61(16):7H–12H.
19. Giner V, Poch E, Bragulat E, et al. Renin-angiotensin system genetic polymorphisms and salt sensitivity in essential hypertension. Hypertension 2000; 35(1 Pt 2):512–7.

20. Poch E, González D, de la Sierra A, et al. Genetic variation of the gamma sub-unit of the epithelial Na+ channel and essential hypertension. Relationship with salt sensitivity. Am J Hypertens 2000;13(6 Pt 1):648–53.

21. Poch E, González D, Giner V, et al. Molecular basis of salt sensitivity in human hypertension. Evaluation of renin-angiotensin-aldosterone system gene polymorphisms. Hypertension 2001;38(5):1204–9.

22. Caprioli J, Mele C, Mossali C, et al. Polymorphisms of EDNRB, ATG, and ACE genes in salt-sensitive hypertension. Can J Physiol Pharmacol 2008;86(8):505–10.

23. Dengel DR, Brown MD, Ferrell RE, et al. Role of angiotensin converting enzyme genotype in sodium sensitivity in older hypertensives. Am J Hypertens 2001;14(12):1178–84.

24. Luft FC, Weinberger MH, Fineberg NS, et al. Effects of age on renal sodium homeostasis and its relevance to sodium sensitivity. Am J Med 1987;82(1B):9–15.

25. Anderson DE, Fedorova OV, Morrell CH, et al. Endogenous sodium pump inhibitors and age-associated increases in salt sensitivity of blood pressure in normotensives. Am J Physiol Regul Integr Comp Physiol 2008;294(4):R1248–54.

26. Hernandez Schulman I, Raij L. Salt sensitivity and hypertension after menopause: role of nitric oxide and angiotensin II. Am J Nephrol 2006;26(2):170–80.

27. Coylewright M, Reckelhoff JF, Ouyang P. Menopause and hypertension: an age-old debate. Hypertension 2008;51(4):952–9.

28. Fang CC, Chen YM, Chu TS, et al. Correlation between renin responsiveness to furosemide and antihypertensive effect of captopril in patients with normal-renin essential hypertension. J Formos Med Assoc 1993;92(11):937–41.

29. Garcia Zozaya JL, Padilla Viloria M, Rodriguez L, et al. The renin-angiotensin-aldosterone system in normal elderly subjects. Res Commun Chem Pathol Pharmacol 1983;40(2):289–99.

30. Weidmann P, De Myttenaere-Bursztein S, Maxwell MH, et al. Effect on aging on plasma renin and aldosterone in normal man. Kidney Int 1975;8(5):325–33.

31. Wilson TW, McCaulay FA, Waslen TA. Effects of aging on responses to furosemide. Prostaglandins 1989;38(6):675–87.

32. Yavuz BB, Yavuz B, Tayfur O, et al. White coat effect and its clinical implications in the elderly. Clin Exp Hypertens 2009;31(4):306–15.

33. Staessen JA, Fagard R, Thijs L, et al. Randomised double-blind comparison of placebo and active treatment for older patients with isolated systolic hypertension. The Systolic Hypertension in Europe (Syst-Eur) Trial Investigators. Lancet 1997;350(9080):757–64.

34. Safar H, Chahwakilian A, Boudali Y, et al. Arterial stiffness, isolated systolic hypertension, and cardiovascular risk in the elderly. Am J Geriatr Cardiol 2006;15(3):178–82 [quiz: 83].

35. Franklin SS, Jacobs MJ, Wong ND, et al. Predominance of isolated systolic hypertension among middle-aged and elderly US hypertensives: analysis based on National Health and Nutrition Examination Survey (NHANES) III. Hypertension 2001;37(3):869–74.

36. Izzo JL, Levy D, Black HR. Clinical Advisory Statement. Importance of systolic blood pressure in older Americans. Hypertension 2000;35(5):1021–4.

37. Young JH, Klag MJ, Muntner P, et al. Blood pressure and decline in kidney function: findings from the Systolic Hypertension in the Elderly Program (SHEP). J Am Soc Nephrol 2002;13(11):2776–82.

38. Pini R, Cavallini MC, Palmieri V, et al. Central but not brachial blood pressure predicts cardiovascular events in an unselected geriatric population: the ICARe Dicomano Study. J Am Coll Cardiol 2008;51(25):2432–9.

39. Pickering TG, Davidson K, Gerin W, et al. Masked hypertension. Hypertension 2002;40(6):795–6.

40. Bobrie G, Chatellier G, Genes N, et al. Cardiovascular prognosis of "masked hypertension" detected by blood pressure self-measurement in elderly treated hypertensive patients. JAMA 2004;291(11):1342–9.

41. Björklund K, Lind L, Zethelius B, et al. Isolated ambulatory hypertension predicts cardiovascular morbidity in elderly men. Circulation 2003;107(9): 1297–302.

42. Cacciolati C, Hanon O, Alpérovitch A, et al. Masked hypertension in the elderly: cross-sectional analysis of a population-based sample. Am J Hypertens 2011; 24(6):674–80.

43. Johnson AG. NSAIDs and blood pressure. Clinical importance for older patients. Drugs Aging 1998;12(1):17–27.

44. Applegate WB, Davis BR, Black HR, et al. Prevalence of postural hypotension at baseline in the Systolic Hypertension in the Elderly Program (SHEP) cohort. J Am Geriatr Soc 1991;39(11):1057–64.

45. Conen D, Chae CU, Guralnik JM, et al. Influence of blood pressure and blood pressure change on the risk of congestive heart failure in the elderly. Swiss Med Wkly 2010;140(13–14):202–8.

46. Cushman WC, Evans GW, Byington RP, et al. Effects of intensive blood-pressure control in type 2 diabetes mellitus. N Engl J Med 2010;362(17):1575–85.

47. Denardo SJ, Gong Y, Nichols WW, et al. Blood pressure and outcomes in very old hypertensive coronary artery disease patients: an INVEST substudy. Am J Med 2010;123(8):719–26.

48. Appel LJ, Espeland MA, Easter L, et al. Effects of reduced sodium intake on hypertension control in older individuals: results from the Trial of Nonpharmacologic Interventions in the Elderly (TONE). Arch Intern Med 2001;161(5):685–93.

49. Ruixing Y, Weixiong L, Hanjun Y, et al. Diet, lifestyle, and blood pressure of the middle-aged and elderly in the Guangxi Bai Ku Yao and Han populations. Am J Hypertens 2008;21(4):382–7.

50. Whelton PK, Appel LJ, Espeland MA, et al. Sodium reduction and weight loss in the treatment of hypertension in older persons: a randomized controlled trial of nonpharmacologic interventions in the elderly (TONE). TONE Collaborative Research Group. JAMA 1998;279(11):839–46.

51. National Institute for Health and Care Excellence (NICE). Hypertension: management of hypertension in adults in primary care. 2006. Available at: http://www.nice.org.uk/CG034. Accessed March 2013.

52. Prevention of stroke by antihypertensive drug treatment in older persons with isolated systolic hypertension. Final results of the Systolic Hypertension in the Elderly Program (SHEP). SHEP Cooperative Research Group. JAMA 1991; 265(24):3255–64.

53. Dhalla IA, Gomes T, Yao Z, et al. Chlorthalidone versus hydrochlorothiazide for the treatment of hypertension in older adults: a population-based cohort study. Ann Intern Med 2013;158(6):447–55.

54. Major outcomes in high-risk hypertensive patients randomized to angiotensin-converting enzyme inhibitor or calcium channel blocker vs diuretic: the Antihypertensive and Lipid-Lowering Treatment to Prevent Heart Attack Trial (ALLHAT). JAMA 2002;288(23):2981–97.

55. Mancia G, Brown M, Castaigne A, et al. Outcomes with nifedipine GITS or Co-amilozide in hypertensive diabetics and nondiabetics in Intervention as a Goal in Hypertension (INSIGHT). Hypertension 2003;41(3):431–6.

56. Messerli FH, Grossman E, Goldbourt U. Are beta-blockers efficacious as first-line therapy for hypertension in the elderly? A systematic review. JAMA 1998; 279(23):1903–7.

57. Barzilay JI, Davis BR, Cutler JA, et al. Fasting glucose levels and incident diabetes mellitus in older nondiabetic adults randomized to receive 3 different classes of antihypertensive treatment: a report from the Antihypertensive and Lipid-Lowering Treatment to Prevent Heart Attack Trial (ALLHAT). Arch Intern Med 2006;166(20):2191–201.

58. Wright JT, Probstfield JL, Cushman WC, et al. ALLHAT findings revisited in the context of subsequent analyses, other trials, and meta-analyses. Arch Intern Med 2009;169(9):832–42.

59. Jamerson K, Weber MA, Bakris GL, et al. Benazepril plus amlodipine or hydrochlorothiazide for hypertension in high-risk patients. N Engl J Med 2008; 359(23):2417–28.

60. Ferrario C, Strawn W. Role of the renin-angiotensin-aldosterone system and proinflammatory mediators in cardiovascular disease. Am J Cardiol 2006; 98(1):121–8.

61. Rüster C, Wolf G. Renin-angiotensin-aldosterone system and progression of renal disease. J Am Soc Nephrol 2006;17(11):2985–91.

62. Abdel-Rahman E, Abadir P, Siragy H. Regulation of renal 12(S)-hydroxyeicosatetraenoic acid in diabetes by angiotensin AT1 and AT2 receptors. Am J Physiol Regul Integr Comp Physiol 2008;295(5):R1473–8.

63. Brenner BM, Cooper ME, de Zeeuw D, et al. Effects of losartan on renal and cardiovascular outcomes in patients with type 2 diabetes and nephropathy. N Engl J Med 2001;345(12):861–9.

64. Berl T, Hunsicker LG, Lewis JB, et al. Cardiovascular outcomes in the Irbesartan Diabetic Nephropathy Trial of patients with type 2 diabetes and overt nephropathy. Ann Intern Med 2003;138(7):542–9.

65. Ruggenenti P, Perna A, Remuzzi G. Nefrologia GIdSEi. ACE inhibitors to prevent end-stage renal disease: when to start and why possibly never to stop: a post hoc analysis of the REIN trial results. Ramipril Efficacy in Nephropathy. J Am Soc Nephrol 2001;12(12):2832–7.

66. Turgut F, Balogun RA, Abdel-Rahman EM. Renin-angiotensin-aldosterone system blockade effects on the kidney in the elderly: benefits and limitations. Clin J Am Soc Nephrol 2010;5(7):1330–9.

67. Verdecchia P, Calvo C, Möckel V, et al. Safety and efficacy of the oral direct renin inhibitor aliskiren in elderly patients with hypertension. Blood Press 2007;16(6): 381–91.

68. Mancia G, De Backer G, Dominiczak A, et al. 2007 guidelines for the management of arterial hypertension: the Task Force for the management of arterial hypertension of the European Society of hypertension (ESH) and of the European Society of Cardiology (ESC). J Hypertens 2007;25(6):1105–87.

69. Hunt SA, American College of Cardiology, American Heart Association Task Force on Practice Guidelines, American College of Chest Physicians; International Society for Heart, and Lung Transplantation, Heart Rhythm Society. ACC/AHA 2005 guideline update for the diagnosis and management of chronic heart failure in the adult: a report of the American College of Cardiology/American Heart Association Task Force on Practice Guidelines (Writing Committee to

Update the 2001 Guidelines for the Evaluation and Management of Heart Failure). J Am Coll Cardiol 2005;46(6):e1–82.

70. Winkelmayer WC, Zhang Z, Shahinfar S, et al. Efficacy and safety of angiotensin II receptor blockade in elderly patients with diabetes. Diabetes Care 2006; 29(10):2210–7.

71. Bakris GL, Sarafidis PA, Weir MR, et al, ACCOMPLISH Trial investigators. Renal outcomes with different fixed-dose combination therapies in patients with hypertension at high risk for cardiovascular events (ACCOMPLISH): a prespecified secondary analysis of a randomised controlled trial. Lancet 2010;375(9721): 1173–81.

72. Medical Research Council trial of treatment of hypertension in older adults: principal results. MRC Working Party. BMJ 1992;304(6824):405–12.

73. Messerli FH, Grossman E. beta-Blockers in hypertension: is carvedilol different? Am J Cardiol 2004;93(9A):7B–12B.

74. Fleg JL, Aronow WS, Frishman WH. Cardiovascular drug therapy in the elderly: benefits and challenges. Nat Rev Cardiol 2011;8(1):13–28.

Chronic Kidney Disease in the Elderly

Thin Thin Maw, MBBS, MS[a], Linda Fried, MD, MPH[a,b],*

KEYWORDS

- Elderly • Geriatric • Chronic kidney disease • Renal function • Dialysis

KEY POINTS

- The new chronic kidney disease (CKD) classification adds proteinuria and cause of CKD to the definition (Comprehensive Geriatric Assessment: cause, glomerular filtration rate, and albuminuria).
- The CKD-EPI formula decreases the number of younger individuals classified as having CKD, but can increase the number of older individuals. The presence of CKD can be confirmed using cystatin C.
- Older individuals with CKD are more likely to die before progression to end-stage renal disease; they are also at increased risk for cardiovascular disease and a decrease in cognitive and physical function.
- The target blood pressure for CKD is less than 140/90 mm Hg in nonproteinuric patients and less than 130/80 mm Hg in proteinuric patients.
- Tight glucose control is not recommended in type 2 diabetes with CKD.

INTRODUCTION

The elderly population in developed countries has been growing because of the decline of mortality and the increased number of "baby boomers". In the United States, it is estimated that there will be a 19.6% increase (71 million) in individuals older than 65 years by 2030 and that by 2050, 1 in 5 adults will be older than 65 years.[1,2] The risk factors for chronic kidney disease (CKD) (eg, hypertension and diabetes) increase in prevalence in the elderly, and the effect of the risk factors is cumulative over many years. As a result, there has been a tremendous increase in the number of elderly patients with CKD and end-stage kidney disease. According to the United States Renal Data System, older adults over 65 years encompass the most rapidly growing subset of the end-stage renal disease (ESRD) population.[3,4]

[a] Renal-Electrolyte Division, University of Pittsburgh School of Medicine, 3550 Terrace Street, Pittsburgh, PA 15261, USA; [b] Renal Section, VA Pittsburgh Healthcare System, University Drive, Mailstop 111F-U, Pittsburgh, PA 15240, USA
* Corresponding author.
E-mail address: linda.fried@va.gov

Clin Geriatr Med 29 (2013) 611–624
http://dx.doi.org/10.1016/j.cger.2013.05.003
0749-0690/13/$ – see front matter Published by Elsevier Inc.

The National Health and Nutrition Examination Survey (NHANES) compared the prevalence of nondialysis-requiring CKD from 1988 to 1994, and from 1994 to 2004, in noninstitutionalized civilians.[5] There was a significant increase in the prevalence of CKD from 10.3% to 13.1% of the population, with the greatest percentage increase in those older than 70 years of age, rising from a prevalence of 37% to 47%.[6]

The combination of high prevalence and often subclinical disease can be controversial. Some argue that CKD is an underrecognized epidemic with increasing prevalence and incidence, particularly in older adults, which is associated with excess risk to their renal and cardiovascular health, physical functioning, and mortality. Others claim that the relatively recent standardized definitions of CKD have had the unintended consequence of exaggerating the prevalence, because (1) the definitions do not adequately separate CKD (disease) from normal renal senescence, and (2) the formulas used to define CKD have not been well validated in the elderly, and may misclassify many older individuals as having CKD when they do not.

DEFINITIONS AND STAGING OF CHRONIC KIDNEY DISEASE

In 2002, the National Kidney Foundation Kidney Disease Outcomes Quality Initiative (KDOQI) published a clinical practice guideline to standardize the definition of CKD and to help guide management, including risk stratification for progression and complications of CKD.[7] CKD was defined by the reduction of glomerular filtration rate (GFR) to less than 60 mL/min/1.73 m^2 and/or evidence of kidney damage, such as proteinuria (albuminuria >30 mg/g of creatinine), glomerular-based or tubular-based hematuria (not urologic), or abnormal renal imaging and pathologic abnormalities of 3 months' duration or longer, irrespective of the cause. The severity of CKD was classified in 5 stages, with 1 being evidence of kidney damage without a decrease in estimated GFR (eGFR) and stage 5 being ESRD (**Table 1**). For this definition, GFR is typically estimated by a formula (**Table 2**). Twenty-four-hour urine creatinine clearance can be used, but is cumbersome and often inaccurate because of difficulties in obtaining a full collection. Measured GFR is not readily available clinically, although it may available in certain situations. GFR is typically estimated using the Modification of Diet in Renal Disease (MDRD) formula. This equation was developed from a cohort of 1628 patients with a GFR lower than 60 mL/min/1.73 m^2 who were enrolled in the MDRD study.[8] This formula contains age, race, and serum creatinine. The age, race, and gender are required as creatinine generation changes with muscle mass, and is lower in women, whites, and older individuals.

Table 1
Stages of CKD in KDOQI

	eGFR (mL/min/1.73 m^2)		Marker of Kidney Damage[a]
Stage 1	≥90	Normal to high	Present
Stage 2	60–89	Mild	Present
Stage 3	30–59	Moderate	Not required
Stage 4	15–29	Severe	Not required
Stage 5	<15 or dialysis	Kidney failure	Not required

[a] Kidney damage is referred to as pathologic abnormalities or markers of damage, including abnormalities in blood or urine tests or imaging studies.

Data from National Kidney Foundation. K/DOQI clinical practice guidelines for chronic kidney disease: evaluation, classification, and stratification. Am J Kidney Dis 2002;39(2 Suppl 1):S1–266.

Table 2
Formulas to measure renal function

Name	Patient Type	Equation
Cockcroft-Gault	All	$C_{Cr} = [(140 - age) \times weight]/(72 \times S_{Cr}) \times 0.85$ (if patient is female)
MDRD	All	$GFR = 186 \times (S_{Cr})^{-1.154} \times (age)^{-0.203} \times 0.742$ (if patient is female) or $\times 1.212$ (if patient is black)
MDRD adjusted	All	$GFR = 175 \times (standardized\ S_{Cr})^{-1.154} \times (age)^{-0.203} \times 0.742$ (if patient is female) or $\times 1.212$ (if patient is black)
CKD-EPI	Women: Creatinine level ≤0.7 mg/dL	
	White women	$eGFR = 144 \times (S_{Cr}/0.7)^{-0.329} \times (0.993)^{Age}$
	Black women	$eGFR = 166 \times (S_{Cr}/0.7)^{-0.329} \times (0.993)^{Age}$
	Women: Creatinine level >0.7 mg/dL	
	White women	$eGFR = 144 \times (S_{Cr}/0.7)^{-1.209} \times (0.993)^{Age}$
	Black women	$eGFR = 166 \times (S_{Cr}/0.7)^{-1.209} \times (0.993)^{Age}$
	Men: Creatinine level ≤0.9 mg/dL	
	White men	$eGFR = 141 \times (S_{Cr}/0.9)^{-0.411} \times (0.993)^{Age}$
	Black men	$eGFR = 163 \times (S_{Cr}/0.9)^{-0.411} \times (0.993)^{Age}$
	Women: Creatinine level >0.9 mg/dL	
	White men	$eGFR = 141 \times (S_{Cr}/0.9)^{-1.209} \times (0.993)^{Age}$
	Black men	Black man: $eGFR = 163 \times (S_{Cr}/0.9)^{-1.209} \times (0.993)^{Age}$
Cystatin C[11]	Cystatin C alone	$eGFR = 76.7 \times (cystatin\ C)^{-1.18}$
	CKD-EPI Cystatin	$eGFR = 127.7 \times (cystatin\ C)^{-1.17} \times (age)^{-0.13} \times (0.91$ if patient is female) $\times$ (1.06 if patient is black)
	Combined cystatin C and creatinine	$eGFR = 177.6 \times (creatinine)^{-0.65} \times$ $(cystatin\ C\ in\ mg/L)^{-0.57} \times (age)^{-0.20} \times (0.82$ if patient is female) $\times$ (1.11 if patient is black)
Berlin Initiative Study (BIS)[15]	Creatinine alone	$eGFR = 3736 \times creatinine^{-0.87} \times age^{-0.95} \times 0.82$ (if female)
	Combined cystatin C and creatinine	$eGFR = 767 \times (cystatin\ C)^{-0.61} \times creatinine^{-0.40} \times age^{-0.57} \times 0.87$ (if female)

Data from Kidney Disease: Improving Global Outcomes (KDIGO) CKD Work Group. KDIGO 2012 clinical practice guideline for the evaluation and management of chronic kidney disease. Kidney Inter Suppl 2013;3:1–150.

The distribution of normal creatinine values is lower in older individuals, owing to generally lower muscle mass. Therefore in older patients, a creatinine value in the high normal range may actually reflect an abnormal decline in kidney function. Modest change in renal function may be overlooked if there is a concurrent decrease in muscle mass. The formula helps to address this shortcoming of serum creatinine, but it must be noted that the definition of CKD requires persistence. Albuminuria has significant day-to-day variability. eGFR is less variable, but can be affected by factors that affect creatinine generation or hemodynamics. The prevalence of CKD decreases if repeat values are checked.[9]

Since publication of the guideline, several concerns have been raised.[10] There is a concern that the classification overdiagnoses individuals with CKD, which is especially true in the elderly. Later stages (stages 3–5) do not require other evidence of kidney damage. As the eGFR formulas contain age, older individuals are more likely to be classified as stage 3 CKD. Many of these individuals have normal serum creatinine, no albuminuria, and values that are in the range 50 to 60 mL/min/1.73 m². Such values could represent misclassification of CKD. The MDRD formula was derived in a population of individuals with kidney disease. It performs less well in healthier populations, tending to underestimate actual GFR.[11] It was also recognized that stage 3 CKD is broad and that many complications of CKD only occur in those with an eGFR lower than 45 mL/min/1.73 m². Another concern is that patients in earlier stages of CKD with heavy proteinuria but normal GFR are at greater risk of progression than many individuals with stage 3 CKD. Recent studies have found that eGFR and albuminuria are independent risk factors for progression of CKD and other adverse outcomes across the stages of CKD.

These findings have led to an updated classification of stage of CKD by the Kidney Disease Improving Global Outcomes (KDIGO), published in January 2013.[12] Similar to KDOQI, CKD in KDIGO is defined as "abnormalities of kidney structure or function present for >3 months with implications for health." If the abnormalities are present for longer than 3 months, CKD is confirmed. If it is present for less than 3 months, it is not confirmed. The KDIGO classification changes the 1-stage classification to a classification based on cause of kidney disease, GFR category, and albuminuria category (**Table 3**). For the causes of CKD, one first defines whether the kidney disease is related to systemic disease (eg, diabetes or collagen vascular disease), and then to the presumed or observed location of the anatomic or pathologic changes in the kidney (eg, glomerular, tubulointerstitial, vascular [including hypertension], cystic, and congenital). For the GFR stages G1 and G2 the presence of other markers of kidney damage is required to be considered CKD (as for KDOQI). With the joint consideration of albuminuria and GFR, individuals can be classified for risk of progression (**Table 4**). The KDIGO guideline does not combine the eGFR and albuminuria into one classification, as some complications (eg, anemia, bone disease) are more closely related to GFR, and other outcomes may be more closely related to albuminuria.

Table 3
KDIGO classification of CKD

GFR Stages	GFR (mL/min/1.73 m²)	Terms
G1	>90	Normal or high
G2	60–89	Mildly decreased
G3a	45–59	Mildly to moderately decreased
G3b	30–44	Moderately to severely decreased
G4	15–29	Severely decreased
G5	<15	Kidney failure

Albuminuria Stages	AER or ACR (mg/24 h or mg/g)	Terms
A1	<30	Normal to mildly increased
A2	30–299	Moderately increased
A3	≥300	Severely increased

Abbreviations: ACR, albumin-to-creatinine ratio; AER, albumin excretion rate (24 hours).
Causes of CKD
1. Presence or absence of systemic disease and
2. Location within kidney of observed or presumed pathologic-anatomic findings such as glomerular diseases, tubulointerstitial diseases, vascular diseases, cystic and congenital diseases.
Data from Kidney Disease: Improving Global Outcomes (KDIGO) CKD Work Group. KDIGO 2012 clinical practice guideline for the evaluation and management of chronic kidney disease. Kidney Inter Suppl 2013;3:1–150.

Table 4
Risk of progression of CKD (KDIGO)

Level of Risk	Staging of CKD (G Stages and/or A Stages)
Low risk	G1 or G2 with A1
Moderately increased risk	G1 or G2 with A2 G3a with A1
High risk	G1 or G2 with A3 G3a with A2 G3b with A1
Very high risk	G3a with A3 G3b with A2 or A3 G4 or G5 with any level of A

G stages: level of eGFR (see **Table 2**).
 A Stages: level of albuminuria (see **Table 2**).
 Data from Kidney Disease: Improving Global Outcomes (KDIGO) CKD Work Group. KDIGO 2012 clinical practice guideline for the evaluation and management of chronic kidney disease. Kidney Inter Suppl 2013;3:1–150.

The KDIGO guideline did not explicitly recommend a specific formula as part of the stated guideline, although the discussion tended to recommend the new Chronic Kidney Disease Epidemiology Collaboration (CKD-EPI) formula. The CKD-EPI formula was developed using a consortium of 16 studies that included both measured GFR and creatinine values. The CKD-EPI equation was developed in an attempt to lessen the systematic underestimation of GFR seen at higher levels of renal function with MDRD. A recent meta-analysis by Earley and colleagues[13] found that the CKD-EPI formula was more accurate and less biased in studies where the mean measured GFR was higher (>60 mL/min/1.73 m^2), whereas the MDRD formula was more accurate in those with lower GFR (CKD studies). This dichotomy generally means that CKD-EPI is less likely to diagnose an individual with CKD. However, this is not the case in the elderly. In those older than 70 years, the CKD-EPI formula tends to classify more individuals as having CKD (**Fig. 1**).[14] In the Berlin Initiative Study (BIS), new formulas were derived in 610 individuals older than 70 (mean age 78.5) years.[15] The

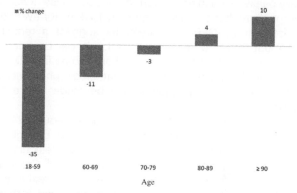

Fig. 1. Change in proportion with CKD stage 3 or worse by age using the CKD-EPI formula rather than the MDRD formula. (*Data from* Schold JD, Navaneethan SD, Jolly SE, et al. Implications of the CKD-EPI GFR estimation equation in clinical practice. Clin J Am Soc Nephrol 2011;6(3):497–504.)

best formula contained cystatin C and creatinine, although a formula was also derived with creatinine alone. The formulas were more accurate in comparison with prior formulas, but still required validation in an external sample. In addition, the study sample was entirely Caucasians, and validation in a more heterogeneous population is necessary.

The misclassification of CKD tends to be in the stage 3a range of eGFR. One approach that may help define who has CKD is to use cystatin C as a confirmation measure. Cystatin C is an endogenous protein (cysteine proteinase inhibitor), like creatinine, but is constitutively produced by all nucleated cells, freely filtered, reabsorbed, and catabolized by the proximal tubules.[16] Most studies have shown that serum cystatin C levels correlate better with GFR than does serum creatinine alone, especially at higher levels of GFR. Cystatin C is not dependent on muscle mass and is less affected than creatinine by race, gender, and age; however, its levels may be influenced by thyroid disease, steroid use, and inflammation. Cystatin C has a more linear relationship with the risk of adverse events such as cardiovascular disease or mortality than does serum creatinine or creatinine-based eGFR, which shows either a threshold below 60 mL/min/1.73^2 or a U-shaped relationship with very low creatinine or eGFR values showing an increased risk.[17] This likely relates to the loss of muscle with disease, leading to decreased creatinine generation and an artificially high eGFR. There are formulas generated to estimate GFR based on cystatin C alone or a combined cystatin C and creatinine equation. This latter equation may be the most accurate at estimating true GFR.[18] Although cystatin C may not yet be widely available, there are tests approved by the Food and Drug Administration for clinical use, and its availability is expected to increase.

This development has led to a 2-step approach to using creatinine and cystatin C in an attempt to reduce the misclassification of CKD. KDIGO suggested that in individuals with stage 3a GFR but no other markers of kidney damage, a cystatin-based eGFR be calculated. If the cystatin C eGFR (or cystatin C with creatinine eGFR) is greater than 60, CKD is not confirmed. A study by Peralta and colleagues[19] found that the proportion of individuals who are reclassified using this approach is greater in older individuals.

PROGRESSION OF CKD WITH AGE

The GFR generally peaks in the third and fourth decades of life at about 140 mL/min/1.73 m^2, then drops thereafter by about 8 mL/min/1.73 m^2 for every decade of life.[7] Estimates from iothalamate GFR measurements suggest a reduction beginning from the age of about 20 to 30 years by 4.6 mL/min per decade in men and by 7.1 mL/min in women. Based on these observations, some investigators have suggested that renal decline is a natural and not a pathologic phenomenon that occurs with age, and that careful consideration should be made before declaring older patients as CKD patients.

The Baltimore Longitudinal Study of Aging obtained regular 24-hour creatinine clearance over time in individuals without history of kidney or urologic disease or cardiovascular disease, and who had normal glucose tolerance test, urinalysis, and were not receiving treatment with antihypertensives or diuretics.[20] Creatinine generation was lower in older individuals, although the average serum creatinine values did not change, thus indicating that the average clearance declined with age (**Table 5**). Over time, individuals lost clearance; this was especially true in individuals with systolic hypertension.[20,21] However, the decline with age was an average. Across the spectrum of age, in healthy individuals there was a significant subset that did not

Table 5 Kidney function by age				
Age (y)	Creatinine (mg/dL)	Creatinine Excretion (mg/24 h)	CrCl (Baseline) (mL/min/1.73 m²)	Slope (mL/min/1.73 m²/y)
25–34	0.81 ± 0.03	1862 ± 31	140.1 ± 2.5	−1.09 ± 0.70
35–44	0.81 ± 0.01	1746 ± 24	132.6 ± 1.8	−0.11 ± 0.36
45–54	0.83 ± 0.01	1689 ± 18	126.8 ± 1.4	−0.73 ± 0.30
55–64	0.84 ± 0.01	1580 ± 22	119.9 ± 1.7	−1.64 ± 0.41
65–74	0.83 ± 0.01	1409 ± 25	109.5 ± 2.0	−1.30 ± 0.57
75–84	0.84 ± 0.02	1259 ± 45	96.9 ± 2.9	−1.07 ± 0.77
Overall			140.4 ± 4.6	−0.90 ± 0.18

Data from Rowe JW, Andres R, Tobin JD, et al. The effect of age on creatinine clearance in men: a cross-sectional and longitudinal study. J Gerontol 1976;31(2):155–63.

experience a decline with age. Therefore although there is a decline with age, it varies tremendously between individuals.

MANAGEMENT OF RISK FACTORS FOR PROGRESSION OF CKD

The most common risk factors for CKD are diabetes (the most common cause of CKD in the United States) and hypertension.[3] Both of these conditions are more common in older populations than in younger ones. Longer duration and poorer control of either of these conditions predispose greater risk for CKD. Other risk factors include obesity, smoking, hyperuricemia, dyslipidemia, cardiovascular disease, and a family history of renal disease. Certain conditions such as heart failure or cancers that are more prevalent in elders predispose individuals at risk for CKD. Diabetes, proteinuria, and poorly controlled hypertension are all strongly associated with more rapid progression of renal disease and, therefore, management should be focused on these issues.[22]

Hypertension

Hypertension, particularly systolic hypertension, is one of the strongest risk factors for CKD. In the Systolic Hypertension in the Elderly Program, systolic blood pressure (BP) was the strongest BP component that predicted a decline in kidney function, defined as a change in serum creatinine of 0.4 mg/dL at 5 years of follow-up.[23] The risk increased linearly across systolic BP quartiles. The target BP in individuals with CKD is controversial.

The Joint National Committee on Prevention, Detection, Evaluation, and Treatment of High Blood Pressure (JNC 7),[24] the American Diabetes Association, and the prior KDOQI guidelines recommended a target BP of less than 130/80 mm Hg in individuals with CKD. This figure is being reevaluated. Both the MDRD study and the African American Study of Kidney Disease and Hypertension (AASK) evaluated lower BP targets (mean arterial pressure <92 mm Hg) in CKD and did not find that a lower BP target slowed progression of kidney disease overall.[25,26] However, individuals with proteinuria (with what would be A3 in the new KDIGO classification) did benefit from lower BP. It is anticipated that JNC VIII will no longer have the lower BP goal for CKD, although the data support lower BP in those who are proteinuric.

As part of the CKD guidelines, the KDIGO also made a BP recommendation to slow progression of kidney disease,[12] recommending a target BP of 140/90 mm Hg or less if albuminuria is less than 30 mg/d and a BP of 130/80 mm Hg or less if albuminuria is

30 mg/d or greater. One caveat is that the risk of tight target BP control should be considered especially in older adults who are prone to have symptomatic postural hypotension.

In individuals with albuminuria, the recommended antihypertensives should include an angiotensin-converting enzyme inhibitor (ACEI) or angiotensin receptor blocker (ARB). The most common disease that will cause proteinuric kidney disease in the elderly is diabetes, although macroalbuminuric proteinuric kidney disease is still present in a minority of individuals with type 2 diabetes and CKD.[27] There are concerns that the data for the benefit of ACEIs or ARBs in older individuals with CKD is sparse.[28,29] Many studies did not include many older individuals or did not present age-stratified analyses. The RENAAL study, a randomized controlled study of losartan in individuals with type 2 diabetes and proteinuria, found that the use of losartan decreased the risk of ESRD by 50% in individuals older than 65 years.[30] There were no significant differences in the efficacy, rate of medication discontinuation, or hyperkalemia in those older than 65 when compared with younger individuals. By contrast, in a retrospective cohort study of individuals with an eGFR of less than 60 mL/min/1.73 m^2 who began lisinopril in the Kaiser Permanente Northwest database, increasing age was associated with an increased risk of hyperkalemia (potassium >5.5 mEq/L).[31] In this study, they developed a risk prediction score for hyperkalemia that included age, level of eGFR, presence of diabetes, heart failure, use of potassium supplements, use of potassium-sparing diuretics, and starting dose of lisinopril. In AASK, individuals with hyperkalemia tended to be older, although age was not a significant risk factor and the upper limit of age in the study was 70 years.[32] Overall, the data suggest that at least for overtly proteinuric diabetic kidney disease (urine albumin/creatinine ratio >300 mg/g), blockade of the renin-angiotensin system slows kidney disease, but whether it is associated with greater risk is not clear. It is important to avoid medications that increase the risk of hyperkalemia.

The KDIGO recommended ACEIs or ARBs for all individuals with diabetes and an albuminuria level of 30 mg/d or higher, and for nondiabetics if at least 300 mg/d. If the individual does not have these levels of albuminuria, there are no good data to show that the choice of antihypertensive affects decline in kidney function.[33] It is important to point out, however, that most individuals with CKD and hypertension will require multiple medications. If an individual is proteinuric, the use of a diuretic and/or a low salt diet may help also lower proteinuria.

Diabetes

Diabetes is one of the most common causes of CKD in the United States. Many large studies have investigated whether glycemic control in individuals who have type 2 diabetes prevents microvascular outcomes, including nephropathy, which is usually defined as albuminuria.

In these large control trials, including the United Kingdom Prospective Diabetes Study (UKPDS), the Action to Control Cardiovascular Risk in Diabetes (ACCORD), and the Veteran Affair Diabetes trial, tighter glucose control was associated with less frequent development or progression of microalbuminuria.[34–36] However, none of these studies showed an association between tight glucose control and a lesser decline in GFR. Moreover, the study groups with tighter glycemic control had more frequent episodes of hypoglycemia and more weight gain than those in the conventional group. The mortality rate was also higher in the intensive arm in ACCORD.[35]

Individuals with CKD are more likely to develop hypoglycemia. In a Veterans Affairs study, Moen and colleagues[37] found that individuals with CKD were more likely to develop hypoglycemia (glucose <50 mg/dL) after admission to hospital. The risk was highest in individuals with diabetes and CKD, but was also seen in individuals with CKD but without diabetes (compared with those without CKD or diabetes, the relative risk for hypoglycemia was 1.62 in those with CKD but without diabetes, 4.09 in those with diabetes but without CKD, and 8.43 for those with both). Hypoglycemia is associated an increased risk for mortality, perhaps because of arrhythmias.[37–39] As tight control is not associated with improved outcomes and the risk of hypoglycemia is higher in those with CKD, the recent KDIGO CKD guideline has proposed different hemoglobin A_{1c} targets in those with diabetes and CKD.[12] The recommended hemoglobin A_{1c} level is approximately 7%; however, it should be higher than 7% in those with significant comorbidities or limited life expectancy and a risk of hypoglycemia. Individuals at increased risk for hypoglycemia should not be treated to a hemoglobin A_{1c} level lower than 7%.

Acute Kidney Injury

Acute kidney injury (AKI) is increasingly recognized as a risk factor for both the development of CKD and its progression in the older adult population. Furthermore, CKD is recognized as a risk factor for the development of AKI (acute on chronic disease) relating to decreased renal reserve. Older individuals are at increased risk for AKI, owing to aging-related decreased renal reserve as well as an increased use of medications and procedures that increase the risk of AKI. There is an article covering AKI elsewhere in this issue, so this aspect is not addressed in detail here. However, this condition raises a general issue of medication safety in older individuals. Many medications taken by older individuals are cleared by the kidneys. With relative polypharmacy older individuals are at increased risk for medication-related complications. Attention needs to be paid to avoiding drug interactions and dose adjustment of medications for kidney function. Nonsteroidal anti-inflammatories and cyclooxygenase-2 inhibitors may be a common cause of AKI, and should be avoided in individuals with CKD.

PROGNOSIS OF CKD

Although CKD is more common in older individuals than in younger ones, older individuals are less likely to progress to ESRD, perhaps because of slower progression in some cases (especially stage 3a without albuminuria), but also because more advanced CKD carries a higher risk for mortality before developing ESRD.[40] Rates of both mortality and ESRD increase as GFR declines. The likelihood of developing ESRD before dying is higher with lower eGFR (the closer you are to dialysis). Not surprisingly, for any given eGFR, older individuals are more likely than younger ones to die before ESRD, and the eGFR at which the risk for ESRD is greater than mortality differs between younger and older individuals. In a study of US Veterans, the level of GFR below which the likelihood of ESRD was greater than death was 45 for those 18 to 44 years old versus 15 for those aged 65 to 84. Over the age of 85, the risk of death was always higher than the risk for ESRD.[40] ESRD and preparation for ESRD are covered in an article elsewhere in this issue.

Although older individuals may not progress to ESRD, the presence of CKD increases the risk of other adverse aging-related outcomes.

NONRENAL-RELATED OUTCOMES
Cardiovascular

Patients with CKD are 3 times more likely than those without to be hospitalized for myocardial infarction, stroke, or arrhythmia. In the Cardiovascular Health Study, patients with CKD of stage 3 or more had more than twice the prevalence of coronary artery disease and heart failure than did those without CKD, and they were more than 50% more likely to have hypertension.[41,42] In the Cardiovascular Health Study, the risk of myocardial infarction for those with CKD and microalbuminuria was 2.5 times higher than for older adults who had neither of these comorbidities.[43]

For patients who are 65 years and older, lower levels of renal function are an independent risk factor for de novo and progressive cardiovascular disease, as well as all-cause mortality over 3 years. Even mildly elevated creatinine levels are prevalent in patients older than 65 years, and can independently predict all-cause and cardiovascular mortality, cardiovascular disease, and heart failure, in comparison with older adults who do not have elevated creatinine.[41]

There are few studies that have evaluated interventions to decrease cardiovascular disease in CKD. The SHARP study was a randomized, controlled, double-blind study of simvastatin/ezetimibe in individuals with CKD.[44] Treatment decreased atherosclerotic outcomes by 17%. Prior studies have found that statins are not effective in dialysis patients, but are effective at decreasing events in nondialysis CKD.[45,46]

Cognitive and Physical Function

Individuals with advanced CKD have a high prevalence of cognitive impairment. This risk is most prevalent in dialysis patients, but can be seen in earlier CKD.[47] In addition, albuminuria alone is also a risk factor for cognitive impairment.[48] The pattern of cognitive impairment is consistent with vascular disease, and affects predominantly attention and executive function.[47] In nursing home patients, both CKD and ESRD are associated with declines in memory scores.[4,49] The decline is greater with older age.

Individuals with CKD also have poorer physical function on tests of balance and gait speed. These patients are more likely to be frail and to develop functional impairment on longitudinal studies.[50,51] This frailty increases the risk for developing disability and nursing home placement. Individuals who are nursing home patients and develop ESRD are at particular risk for poor outcomes.[49] Individuals with CKD have lower levels of physical activity,[52] and whether focused exercise programs would improve function should be studied in the future.

Bone Disease

Individuals with ESRD have very high fracture rates, due in large part to metabolic bone disease.[53,54] In CKD, early signs of changes in hormones such as FGF-23 can be seen, followed by declines in $1,25(OH)_2$ vitamin D levels. However, parathyroid hormone levels rise later, and elevated phosphorus levels are late findings. In older individuals with stage 3a CKD and in many with stage 3b CKD, the predominant bone disease is osteoporosis.

Cross-sectionally, stage 3 CKD is not associated with lower bone mineral density (BMD), although it does appear to predict faster bone loss.[55,56] Whether the fracture risk is higher in nondialysis CKD, once the other concomitant risk factors have been adjusted for, is controversial. If low BMD is present, both nondialysis CKD and non-CKD patients are at similar risk for fracture, and should be treated.[57] Most osteoporosis medicines can be used when the clearance is greater than 30 mL/min/1.73 m^2.

WHEN TO REFER TO NEPHROLOGY

Not everyone with CKD needs to be seen by nephrology, and this is particularly true for the older individuals with multiple comorbidities and low expectation of progressing to ESRD. There are recommendations in the KDIGO guideline for referral, which

---

Box 1
Criteria for referral to nephrology for CKD

Nephrotic syndrome

Proteinuria >1 g in nondiabetic individuals

Nonurologic hematuria

Recurrent hyperkalemia

Rapid progression of CKD (decline in eGFR >5 mL/min/y)

eGFR <30 mL/min/1.73 m^2

---

are generally appropriate but too liberal with regard to proteinuria. The KDIGO guidelines recommend that all individuals with persistent albuminuria of greater than 300 mg/d should be referred. In the United States the most common patients with persistent albuminuria of greater than 300 mg/d will be diabetic, and unless there are unusual manifestations (eg, rapid increase in proteinuria or presence of hematuria), individuals with diabetes and nonnephrotic proteinuria, and preserved GFR do not necessarily need to be referred to nephrology. Recommendations for when to refer for CKD are shown in **Box 1**.

SUMMARY

Older individual with CKD are a growing social and economic problem. Even as the new CKD-EPI formula decreases the number of younger individuals classified as having CKD, the number of older individuals with CKD remains high. However, the elderly with CKD are more likely to die before progression to ESRD, and are also at increased risk for cardiovascular disease and decrease in cognitive and physical function. The management of older individuals with CKD is similar to that for the younger population; however, we should be not be too stringent with BP and blood sugar control in the elderly, because elderly patients are more vulnerable to hypotension and hypoglycemia. Older individuals with CKD should be managed by a multidisciplinary approach (geriatrician, palliative care and nephrologist) to achieve a better quality of life.

REFERENCES

1. Centers for Disease Control and Prevention. Public health and aging: trends in aging—United States and worldwide. JAMA 2003;289(11):1371–3.
2. Stevens LA, Coresh J, Levey AS. CKD in the elderly—old questions and new challenges: World Kidney Day 2008. Am J Kidney Dis 2008;51(3):353–7.
3. Collins AJ, Foley RN, Chavers B, et al. United States renal data system 2011 Annual data report: atlas of chronic kidney disease & end-stage renal disease in the United States. Am J Kidney Dis 2012;59(1 Suppl 1):A7, e1–420.
4. Collins AJ, Foley RN, Herzog C, et al. Excerpts from the US renal data system 2009 Annual data report. Am J Kidney Dis 2010;55(1 Suppl 1):S1–420, A6–7.
5. Coresh J, Astor BC, Greene T, et al. Prevalence of chronic kidney disease and decreased kidney function in the adult US population: third National Health and Nutrition Examination Survey. Am J Kidney Dis 2003;41(1):1–12.
6. Coresh J, Selvin E, Stevens LA, et al. Prevalence of chronic kidney disease in the United States. JAMA 2007;298(17):2038–47.

7. National Kidney Foundation. K/DOQI clinical practice guidelines for chronic kidney disease: evaluation, classification, and stratification. Am J Kidney Dis 2002; 39(2 Suppl 1):S1–266.
8. Levey AS, Bosch JP, Lewis JB, et al. A more accurate method to estimate glomerular filtration rate from serum creatinine: a new prediction equation. Modification of Diet in Renal Disease Study Group. Ann Intern Med 1999;130(6):461–70.
9. Brook MO, Bottomley MJ, Mevada C, et al. Repeat testing is essential when estimating chronic kidney disease prevalence and associated cardiovascular risk. QJM 2012;105(3):247–55.
10. Levey AS, de Jong PE, Coresh J, et al. The definition, classification, and prognosis of chronic kidney disease: a KDIGO Controversies Conference report. Kidney Int 2011;80(1):17–28.
11. Rule AD, Larson TS, Bergstrath EJ, et al. Using serum creatinine to estimate glomerular filtration rate: accuracy in good health and in chronic kidney disease. Ann Intern Med 2004;141(12):929–37.
12. Kidney Disease: Improving Global Outcomes (KDIGO) CKD Work Group. KDIGO 2012 clinical practice guideline for the evaluation and management of chronic kidney disease. Kidney Int Suppl 2013;3:1–150.
13. Earley A, Miskulin D, Lamb EJ, et al. Estimating equations for glomerular filtration rate in the era of creatinine standardization: a systematic review. Ann Intern Med 2012;156(11):785–95 W–270, W–271, W–272, W–273, W–274, W–275, W–276, W–277, W–278.
14. Schold JD, Navaneethan JD, Jolly SE, et al. Implications of the CKD-EPI GFR estimation equation in clinical practice. Clin J Am Soc Nephrol 2011;6(3):497–504.
15. Schaeffner ES, Ebert N, Delanaye P, et al. Two novel equations to estimate kidney function in persons aged 70 years or older. Ann Intern Med 2012;157(7):471–81.
16. Randers E, Erlandsen EJ. Serum cystatin C as an endogenous marker of the renal function—a review. Clin Chem Lab Med 1999;37(4):389–95.
17. Shlipak MG, Sarnak MJ, Katz R, et al. Cystatin C and the risk of death and cardiovascular events among elderly persons. N Engl J Med 2005;352(20):2049–60.
18. Inker LA, Schmid CH, Tighiouart H, et al. Estimating glomerular filtration rate from serum creatinine and cystatin C. N Engl J Med 2012;367(1):20–9.
19. Peralta CA, Katz R, Sarnak MJ, et al. Cystatin C identifies chronic kidney disease patients at higher risk for complications. J Am Soc Nephrol 2011;22(1):147–55.
20. Rowe JW, Adres R, Tobin JD, et al. The effect of age on creatinine clearance in men: a cross-sectional and longitudinal study. J Gerontol 1976;31(2):155–63.
21. Lindeman RD, Tobin J, Shock NW. Longitudinal studies on the rate of decline in renal function with age. J Am Geriatr Soc 1985;33(4):278–85.
22. Soares CM, Diniz JS, Lima EM, et al. Predictive factors of progression to chronic kidney disease stage 5 in a predialysis interdisciplinary programme. Nephrol Dial Transplant 2009;24(3):848–55.
23. Young JH, Klag MJ, Muntner P, et al. Blood pressure and decline in kidney function: findings from the Systolic Hypertension in the Elderly Program (SHEP). J Am Soc Nephrol 2002;13(11):2776–82.
24. Chobanian AV, Bakris GL, Black HR, et al. The Seventh report of the joint National Committee on Prevention, Detection, Evaluation, and Treatment of High Blood Pressure: the JNC 7 report. JAMA 2003;289(19):2560–72.

25. Klahr S, Levey AS, Beck GJ, et al. The effects of dietary protein restriction and blood-pressure control on the progression of chronic renal disease. Modification of Diet in Renal Disease Study Group. N Engl J Med 1994;330(13): 877–84.
26. Wright JT Jr, Bakris G, Greene T, et al. Effect of blood pressure lowering and antihypertensive drug class on progression of hypertensive kidney disease: results from the AASK trial. JAMA 2002;288(19):2421–31.
27. Kramer HJ, Nguyen QD, Curhan G, et al. Renal insufficiency in the absence of albuminuria and retinopathy among adults with type 2 diabetes mellitus. JAMA 2003;289(24):3273–7.
28. O'Hare AM, Kaufman JS, Covinsky KE, et al. Current guidelines for using angiotensin-converting enzyme inhibitors and angiotensin II-receptor antagonists in chronic kidney disease: is the evidence base relevant to older adults? Ann Intern Med 2009;150(10):717–24.
29. Weiss JW, Thorp ML, O'Hare AM. Renin-angiotensin system blockade in older adults with chronic kidney disease: a review of the literature. Curr Opin Nephrol Hypertens 2010;19(5):413–9.
30. Winkelmayer WC, Zhang Z, Shahinfar S, et al. Efficacy and safety of angiotensin II receptor blockade in elderly patients with diabetes. Diabetes Care 2006; 29(10):2210–7.
31. Johnson ES, Weinstein JR, Thorp ML, et al. Predicting the risk of hyperkalemia in patients with chronic kidney disease starting lisinopril. Pharmacoepidemiol Drug Saf 2010;19(3):266–72.
32. Weinberg JM, Appel LJ, Bakris G, et al. Risk of hyperkalemia in nondiabetic patients with chronic kidney disease receiving antihypertensive therapy. Arch Intern Med 2009;169(17):1587–94.
33. Rahman M, Ford CE, Cutler JA, et al. Long-term renal and cardiovascular outcomes in Antihypertensive and Lipid-Lowering Treatment to Prevent Heart Attack Trial (ALLHAT) participants by baseline estimated GFR. Clin J Am Soc Nephrol 2012;7(6):989–1002.
34. Duckworth W, Abraira C, Moritz T, et al. Glucose control and vascular complications in veterans with type 2 diabetes. N Engl J Med 2009;360(2):129–39.
35. Gerstein HC, Miller ME, Byington RP, et al. Effects of intensive glucose lowering in type 2 diabetes. N Engl J Med 2008;358(24):2545–59.
36. Patel A, MacMahon S, Chalmers J, et al. Intensive blood glucose control and vascular outcomes in patients with type 2 diabetes. N Engl J Med 2008; 358(24):2560–72.
37. Moen MF, Zhan M, Hsu VD, et al. Frequency of hypoglycemia and its significance in chronic kidney disease. Clin J Am Soc Nephrol 2009;4(6):1121–7.
38. Nordin C. The case for hypoglycaemia as a proarrhythmic event: basic and clinical evidence. Diabetologia 2010;53(8):1552–61.
39. Zoungas S, Patel A, Chalmers J, et al. Severe hypoglycemia and risks of vascular events and death. N Engl J Med 2010;363(15):1410–8.
40. O'Hare AM, Choi AL, Bertenthal D, et al. Age affects outcomes in chronic kidney disease. J Am Soc Nephrol 2007;18(10):2758–65.
41. Fried LF, Shlipak MG, Crump C, et al. Renal insufficiency as a predictor of cardiovascular outcomes and mortality in elderly individuals. J Am Coll Cardiol 2003;41(8):1364–72.
42. Manjunath G, Tighiouart H, Coresh J, et al. Level of kidney function as a risk factor for cardiovascular outcomes in the elderly. Kidney Int 2003;63(3): 1121–9.

43. Rifkin DE, Katz R, Chonchol M, et al. Albuminuria, impaired kidney function and cardiovascular outcomes or mortality in the elderly. Nephrol Dial Transplant 2010;25(5):1560–7.

44. Baigent C, Landray MJ, Reith C, et al. The effects of lowering LDL cholesterol with simvastatin plus ezetimibe in patients with chronic kidney disease (Study of Heart and Renal Protection): a randomised placebo-controlled trial. Lancet 2011;377(9784):2181–92.

45. Palmer SC, Craig JC, Navaneethan SD, et al. Benefits and harms of statin therapy for persons with chronic kidney disease: a systematic review and meta-analysis. Ann Intern Med 2012;157(4):263–75.

46. Upadhyay A, Earley A, Lamont JL, et al. Lipid-lowering therapy in persons with chronic kidney disease: a systematic review and meta-analysis. Ann Intern Med 2012;157(4):251–62.

47. Murray AM. Cognitive impairment in the aging dialysis and chronic kidney disease populations: an occult burden. Adv Chronic Kidney Dis 2008;15(2):123–32.

48. Weiner DE, Bartolomei K, Scott T, et al. Albuminuria, cognitive functioning, and white matter hyperintensities in homebound elders. Am J Kidney Dis 2009;53(3):438–47.

49. Kurella Tamura M, Covinsky KE, Chertow GM, et al. Functional status of elderly adults before and after initiation of dialysis. N Engl J Med 2009;361(16):1539–47.

50. Fried LF, Lee JS, Shlipak M, et al. Chronic kidney disease and functional limitation in older people: health, aging and body composition study. J Am Geriatr Soc 2006;54(5):750–6.

51. Shlipak MG, Stehman-Breen C, Fried LF, et al. The presence of frailty in elderly persons with chronic renal insufficiency. Am J Kidney Dis 2004;43(5):861–7.

52. Johansen KL, Chertow GM, Kutner NG, et al. Low level of self-reported physical activity in ambulatory patients new to dialysis. Kidney Int 2010;78(11):1164–70.

53. Kidney Disease: Improving Global Outcomes (KDIGO) CKD-MBD Work Group. KDIGO clinical practice guideline for the diagnosis, evaluation, prevention, and treatment of Chronic Kidney Disease-Mineral and Bone Disorder (CKD-MBD). Kidney Int Suppl 2009;(113):S1–130.

54. Seiler S, Heine GH, Fliser D. Clinical relevance of FGF-23 in chronic kidney disease. Kidney Int Suppl 2009;(114):S34–42.

55. Fried LF, Shlipak MG, Stehman-Breen C, et al. Kidney function predicts the rate of bone loss in older individuals: the Cardiovascular Health Study. J Gerontol A Biol Sci Med Sci 2006;61(7):743–8.

56. Hsu CY, Cummings SR, McCulloch CE, et al. Bone mineral density is not diminished by mild to moderate chronic renal insufficiency. Kidney Int 2002;61(5):1814–20.

57. Yenchek RH, Ix JH, Shlipak MG, et al. Bone mineral density and fracture risk in older individuals with CKD. Clin J Am Soc Nephrol 2012;7(7):1130–6.

Dialysis Therapies in Older Patients with End-Stage Renal Disease

Tuschar Malavade, MD, DNB, Ahmed Sokwala, MD,
Sarbjit Vanita Jassal, MB, MD, FRCPC*

KEYWORDS

- Hemodialysis • Peritoneal dialysis • Dialysis • Elderly

KEY POINTS

- Mortality and morbidity is maximal in the first 3 months after dialysis initiation.
- The functional and cognitive burden is higher in older patients undergoing chronic dialysis therapy than in age-matched community-dwelling seniors not on dialysis therapy.
- In older patients, hemodialysis may offer minimally longer survival duration than peritoneal dialysis, but this is at the expense of well-being.
- Hemodialysis patients describe high levels of postdialysis fatigue and report a prolonged time to recovery after the dialysis treatment, which can limit activities of daily living.
- Patients undergoing peritoneal dialysis spend less time in hospital or hospital-like environments, and undergo fewer tests and procedures, than those undergoing hemodialysis.

INTRODUCTION

As noted in previous articles, patients with a variety of kidney diseases often develop a picture of progressive scarring and renal dysfunction termed chronic kidney disease (CKD). By definition, all patients with irreversible renal damage that has persisted for at least 3 months are at risk of progressive deterioration. The nomenclature used for advanced renal disease has evolved over the years, and consequently can be confusing; therefore, for the purposes of this article the term end-stage renal disease (ESRD) is used to describe those individuals with CKD Stage 5, or estimated glomerular filtration rate (eGFR) of less than 15 mL/min/1.73 m^2, who are approaching or have started on dialysis therapy or have undergone kidney transplantation.

Division of Nephrology, Department of Medicine, University of Toronto, University Health Network, 200 Elizabeth Street, 8N857, Toronto, Ontario M5G 2K8, Canada
* Corresponding author. University Health Network, 200 Elizabeth Street, 8N-857, Toronto, Ontario M5G 2C4, Canada.
E-mail address: vanita.jassal@uhn.ca

Clin Geriatr Med 29 (2013) 625–639
http://dx.doi.org/10.1016/j.cger.2013.05.005
0749-0690/13/$ – see front matter © 2013 Elsevier Inc. All rights reserved.

Causes of ESRD in Older Patients

Data from renal registries show the leading causes of renal disease in elderly patients starting dialysis are hypertension, vascular disease, and diabetes. Diabetic nephropathy, while common, is less common in those 80 years and older than in younger patients, because of the competing risk of death due to vascular disease. Often a large proportion of elderly patients have "unknown" or unconfirmed causes for their renal disease. Particularly in areas without eGFR reporting, renal disease remains unrecognized and older patients often present late, with insidious symptoms, at a time when the kidneys have become scarred and shrunken. In these cases it is likely that vascular and hypertensive changes may be the major reason for progression to ESRD, as many of these older individuals do have other evidence of diffuse vascular disease. ESRD arising from chronic or repeated obstructive uropathy is more common in the elderly age groups than in those aged 20 to 55 years. Chronic glomerular diseases, vasculitides, and cystic diseases of the kidney, though still important, are less common.[1]

EPIDEMIOLOGY OF ESRD

Among all age groups, the rate of growth in incident dialysis use per million population is highest in those aged 75 years or older.

The number of individuals with kidney disease may increase either because the total population at risk of kidney disease increases (population growth), or because the disease burden has increased. To better understand which factors are at play, the number of patients starting dialysis is often reported as a rate within the population at risk (number of cases per million population). In the dialysis literature, most countries report increasing rates of patients initiating dialysis (incident patients) per million, suggesting a growth in the disease burden. Until the early 2000s, the fastest growth occurred in the rates of patients aged 75 years and older who were started on dialysis, which has resulted in an increase in the median age of the total population on dialysis. In the United Kingdom, the median age of patients starting renal replacement therapy increased from 63.8 years in 1998 to 65.2 years in 2005.[2] However, demographic trends appear to be shifting. In the United States and Canada the median age of patients increased in the early 2000s; however, current United States data show that whereas the adjusted incident rate of ESRD continues to grow (growth rates of 12.2% since 2000 for patients aged 75 and older, to 1773 per million population in 2010), the rates for those aged 65 to 74 are now decreasing (current rates for the age group 65–74 years have fallen to levels that are 3.1% lower in 2010 than in 2000).[3]

Prevalent rates for those aged 75 years or more have also increased, as survival has improved over time. Data from the Dialysis Outcomes and Practice Patterns Study (DOPPS) have shown that although the mean age of study participants increased over time in all DOPPS regions, the uptake of dialysis among elderly individuals varied widely.[4] Belgium, France, and Sweden have the largest populations of individuals aged 75 years and older, with the lowest numbers being seen in Japan. Similar variability is seen across regions in the United States[5] and may reflect differences in the availability of nondialysis care pathways, transplantation rates, and societal expectations.[6,7]

The observed increase in the rate of elderly patients starting dialysis has been largely attributed to aging of the general population; survival and risk of CKD after acute kidney injury; improved survival in patients who have other chronic diseases such as heart failure or cardiovascular disease; increased worldwide dialysis accessibility; and a change in the attitudes of patients and their families, nephrologists, and referring physicians toward the older, frail patient. Hsu and colleagues[8] have shown that the increase in the rate of ESRD over the 20-year period spanning 1976 to 1994 was 70% greater than that seen in CKD rates, suggesting that factors independent of disease prevalence were largely at play. Improved survival rates after acute illness associated with acute kidney injury have been shown to increase the risk of CKD by between 28- and 60-fold.[9,10] Some investigators[11] have previously predicted that upward of 130,000 patients will be started on dialysis in 2015 in the United States alone, although this may be an overestimate, as a wider appreciation of the morbidity associated with dialysis leads to improved access to nondialytic care pathways and fewer older patients being advised to initiate dialysis.

In many centers, in-center hemodialysis (HD) (96%) is the primary treatment used in elderly patients. In Pacific Asia (Taiwan and Hong Kong) and France, peritoneal dialysis (PD) is commonly used in elderly individuals. Statistics show that more than 45% of PD patients in France are aged 75 years or older; however, this number accounts for only 22% of the total number of individuals older than 75 who are starting dialysis. Transplantation remains a relatively infrequently used treatment option for elderly patients with ESRD across most parts of the world, with the highest rates of transplantation in older patients being seen in Norway.

The anticipated survival in those who are started on dialysis is variable, and ranges from several months to years.

- In a recent review, Carson and colleagues elegantly showed how reported survival rates in elderly patients initiated on dialysis vary from several months to years (**Fig. 1**).[12] In Canada the mean life expectancy after dialysis initiation is estimated at 3.2 years (95% confidence interval [CI] 3.0–3.3 years) for those aged between 75 and 79 years at the start of dialysis. In the United States survival rates are lower than in Canada and Europe,[13] likely reflecting the wider use of dialysis therapies in frail or vulnerable patients.

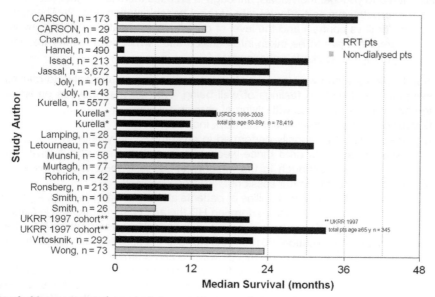

Fig. 1. Mean reported survival for patients aged 65 years or older (unless indicated otherwise) with and without renal replacement therapy (RRT).

- Although not confirmed in all parts of the world, studies from Canada suggest that the overall survival of older patients starting dialysis has improved by 23% (95% CI 20%–27%) over time.[13–15]
- Several studies have shown that the mortality and morbidity seen after dialysis initiation is maximal in the early postdialysis period, with more than one-third of patients dying in the initial 3 months.[16–19]
- In a recent study from Canada, patients aged 75 years or older, or those starting dialysis at a higher residual renal function were more likely to withdraw dialysis early in their treatment course.[19] Particularly in a frail or vulnerable population, this information should be honestly conveyed to both patients and families to allow appropriate decision making.

DOPPS data have shown regional variation in survival, with the median survival being maximal in Japan (median survival duration 5.4 years) and lowest in Australia/New Zealand (estimated at 1.6 years).[4] This variability is likely secondary to differences in comorbidity and selection criteria for dialysis.[7] Several tools are available to estimate survival.[11,13–15] However, these have been derived from population studies, and should only be used to classify patients into groups at high or average risk of mortality. The application of these tools to estimate prognosis and determine treatment at an individual level has not been studied, and some estimate that routine use may result in wrongly placing individuals who may do well into the high-risk category in up to 20% of cases.[20]

Factors influencing survival are similar across all age groups, and include the number and severity of cardiac and vascular comorbidity, cognitive and functional status, markers of inflammation and malnutrition, and the use of venous catheter for access.[18,21–25]

TYPES OF RENAL REPLACEMENT THERAPIES USED IN ELDERLY ESRD PATIENTS

The treatment options available to elderly patients reaching ESRD are identical to those offered to younger individuals, although in practice there is a higher use of non-dialytic care pathways and a lower rate of renal transplantation (**Fig. 2**). The patient phenotype (frail vs nonfrail) and the level of dependency of patient with the involvement of caregiver have to be taken into consideration when deciding the treatment options. Broadly the available options are:

1. Nondialytic care pathway (conservative therapy), using all strategies to minimize symptoms and prolong feelings of well-being. This strategy focuses on limiting the symptoms associated with dying of chronic disease.
2. Dialytic care (renal replacement therapy), including:
   a. In-center HD, traditionally performed in customized dialysis units or hospital-based dialysis units on a thrice-weekly basis. Patients may be involved with some self-care, although in the majority of cases trained staff provides full care during the treatment sessions.
   b. Home HD, performed by families or patients after a period of training. Age itself is not a contraindication to performing HD therapy in the home, and in Canada home nocturnal HD has been used in those aged 65 years or older (Dr C Chan, personal communication, 2013). Although dialysis sessions can be performed daily, many patients perform this between 3 and 5 times a week.
   c. PD, typically offered as a home dialysis modality to individuals who can perform the treatments themselves, or with the assistance of family members. Several centers have inpatient facilities or visiting nurse programs that offer support for those unable to perform self-care PD, and these are discussed in detail later.

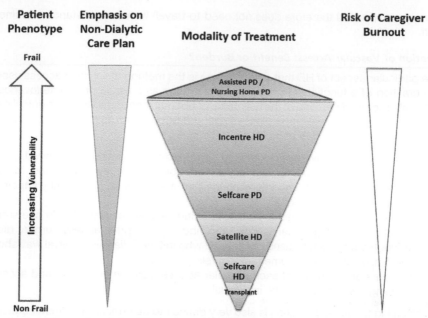

Fig. 2. How the results of the comprehensive geriatric assessment of the patient, and discussion with the caregiver, may influence discussion of modality choice. Discussions about non-dialytic strategies should be initiated in most cases, but a larger degree of emphasis should be placed on those with increased functional or cognitive dependence and on those with higher caregiving needs. HD, hemodialysis; PD, peritoneal dialysis.

d. Hybrid therapy consisting of both HD and PD.
e. Renal transplantation, discussed in subsequent articles elsewhere in this issue. This option is offered to otherwise healthy elderly patients with a low burden of comorbidity and fair life expectancy.

HEMODIALYSIS IN ELDERLY ESRD PATIENTS

The technical aspects of HD in the older population are no different to those in younger individuals. Data from the DOPPS international study, however, suggest that in practice older patients tend to have shorter dialysis treatment times and lower ultrafiltration rates. Despite the shorter sessions, older patients were found to be more likely to meet clinical targets for dialysis dose and phosphate levels. In general, body mass index and weight are lower in older individuals, which, together with the observed lower albumin and phosphate levels, may suggest they are at an increased risk of malnutrition.

HD is most commonly used in older patients because it does not require the patient to be actively involved in the therapy. Patients and families both prefer that it is performed by trained staff in specialized units, but dislike the travel restrictions. In a qualitative questionnaire study, Morton and colleagues[26] found that patients would accept a 2-year reduction in survival to minimize travel restrictions. Although one of the most significant disadvantages of HD is the need to travel to the dialysis center and the time commitment required, HD offers an opportunity for some older patients to have regular social contact with others.[27–29] HD performed within nursing homes or residential settings is a modified form of home dialysis therapy whereby the patient undergoes therapy on-site (and therefore does not need to travel) with the assistance of trained staff.

Creation of Vascular Access: Benefit or Burden?

One particular aspect of HD that differs by age is the method of vascular access used. The creation of a functioning vascular access, such as a fistula or an arteriovenous (AV) graft, is considered one of the hallmarks of optimal renal care. Although guidelines suggest that all individuals regardless of age undergo access assessment, the evaluation of the older patient is particularly challenging.

- Elderly patients have both increased comorbidity and decreased survival.
- Elderly patients experience a higher rate of adverse events related to the procedure; revisions; and interventions that may result in significantly impaired well-being and quality of life.
- Elderly patients might die even before using vascular access.[30–32] In one small report of 37 octogenarians, 32% who had a preemptive access surgery died before the access was used.[31] Of those who initiated dialysis, survival was short and many required placement in a nursing home.
- The risks and benefits of each vascular access must be evaluated, and access planning customized for the individual.

The timing for access creation is also very difficult to determine. Recommendations to consider the fistula as the access of choice, and for all patients to be referred when their eGFR is less than 15 mL/min/1.73 m^2 or when expected to start dialysis in 6 months, may not be the most beneficial or economically viable approach. In the American Society of Nephrology geriatric curriculum, Wright and Danziger[33] question the value of guidelines suggesting that older patients undergo vascular access surgery for fistula or AV graft insertion. The investigators suggest that the creation of a fistula or graft may be futile, as it is unlikely to be used. Vachharajani and colleagues[31] argue that access creation be offered only to those with a life expectancy greater than 180 days, whereas Moist and colleagues[32] argue that fistula creation be limited, among older patients, to those with few comorbidities and a life expectancy on dialysis of longer than 1 to 2 years. These investigators recommend graft use in those with an intermediate life expectancy, and propose that insertion of a semipermanent tunneled line be considered appropriate for those with limited life expectancy starting dialysis therapy.

Studies comparing fistula use across the dialysis population show that fistula use is lower in older individuals, particularly those 75 years or older, in all areas of the world. Patients in Japan had the highest rate of fistula use but also were the most likely to have long-term dialysis therapy, likely because of differences in transplantation policies and practices.[34,35] The reasons for the low rates of fistula use are manifold, but do reflect a higher risk of failure to mature (odds ratio 2.23; 95% CI 1.25–3.96 for those aged 65 years or older[36]) and lower fistula survival rates (5 year cumulative fistula survival rates of 65% vs 71% in those older than and younger than 65 years, respectively[37]).

HOME DIALYSIS IN ELDERLY ESRD PATIENTS

- Home dialysis encompasses both home HD and PD.
- Age is not a contraindication for home HD or PD. In Canada, however, where home HD is promoted, less than 3% of older patients are treated with home HD.[14]

- Older patients do well with PD.[38,39]
- Despite arguments suggesting otherwise, the absolute survival advantage from HD over PD is clinically insignificant,[38] and the quality-of-life benefits greater.[40,41] Data from the French registry for 1613 PD patients aged 75 years or older show a median patient survival of more than 2 years. The median technique survival was unaffected by age and was estimated at 21 months.[39]
- Age has not been found to be a barrier to self-care, although many, possibly wrongly,[42] have attributed the steady decline in the use of PD across the world to self-care barriers. For patients choosing PD, the main advantage is that they are able to integrate their own dialysis treatment schedule into their own lifestyle, allowing them more freedom to pursue personal activities and interests. This aspect is particularly important for older individuals because they are often more dependent on daily routines being followed, and may require more time for simple daily activities.
- While initiation of dialysis places an increased burden on caregivers, the use of PD may also offer caregivers more flexibility to adapt the treatment routines to their circumstances and lifestyle.[26] Under these circumstances it is important to support caregivers, as caregiver stress and burnout may affect rates of technique survival and peritonitis.

Unique Challenges Associated with the Use of Home Dialysis in Older Patients

The 2 most common challenges that older patients face are the need for increased support to manage their own care, and the risk of infection.

Various methods have been used to support elderly patients and caregivers. Home care and nursing home dialysis programs are simple, cost-effective ways of providing dialysis support for the frail older patient.[38] Trained nurses or nursing assistants may help patients or family caregivers appropriately select peritoneal dialysate bag strength, set up cycler machines, or help with some of the daytime continuous ambulatory PD exchanges, blood pressure and weight assessment, or ongoing teaching support.[38,43–46] With the introduction of e-Health technologies, the provision of in-home support will likely continue to improve.

Peritonitis remains one of the most serious complications associated with PD.[47,48] Several smaller studies have suggested that older patients are at higher risk of peritonitis,[47–50] although more recent, larger studies have suggested that the rate of peritonitis is not age dependent.[51,52] Peritonitis treatments are similar, and the episodes themselves seem to resolve as quickly in those older than 70 years as in younger patients.[52] The outcomes, however, are more severe, and observational data suggest that older patients are at 2-fold higher risk of death in the period after peritonitis compared with younger patients.[52]

Using prospectively collected data from 4247 incidental PD patients, Nessim and colleagues[52] found that older patients had a lower rate of gram-positive catheter infections, in particular *Staphylococcus aureus* catheter infections. Two striking observations made included a trend toward lower rates of *S aureus* peritonitis rates in those older than 70 years (rate ratio, 0.93 per decade increase) in more recent years, and no additional risk of gram-negative infections in the older age groups as had been expected.[52] It is now believed that strategies (such as topical mupirocin, luer-lock connectology, and "flush before fill" systems) that target infections associated with touch contamination may differentially benefit the older patient rather than the younger patient, because of age-related changes in dexterity.

COMORBIDITIES ASSOCIATED WITH DIALYSIS TREATMENT IN GERIATRIC PATIENTS

Several studies have suggested that dialysis initiation may exacerbate, or cause, functional and/or cognitive decline (**Fig. 3**). Three recent studies have shown a decline in function among elderly patients at or around the time of dialysis initiation in both those initiating PD and those starting on HD.[16,53,54] A single-center study of patients who initiated dialysis between 2000 and 2005 when aged 80 years or older found that more than 30% of patients experienced functional loss within 6 months.[53] In those starting peritoneal dialysis, 32.5% required either professional caregiver support or transfer to a nursing home.[53] Similarly, elderly nursing home patients experienced a sharp permanent decline in functional status over a 3-month period after starting chronic dialysis therapy.[16] This burden of early functional decline is reflected in the high rates of functional disability and frailty seen in prevalent dialysis patients.[55,56]

The cause of the increased burden of functional decline is unclear. Patients undergoing HD thrice weekly experience a postdialysis recovery period characterized by a profound fatigue. This fatigue, or "time to recover," can vary in duration, but has been noted in some patients to last until the next dialysis session.[57,58] During this time patients report feeling too tired to perform their normal activities; as time progresses the chronicity of the symptoms may alter the family dynamics, and the patient may develop a "learned helplessness."[59] In a survey completed by 100 HD patients of all ages, fatigue on dialysis days and fatigue on nondialysis days were reported by 67% and 40% of patients, respectively.[60] This fatigue may be a significant barrier to physical activity, and contribute to muscle dysfunction and disability.

One of the less appreciated complications of HD that may contribute to functional decline is the effect of forced immobility. The long time during which patients are sitting relatively still in the dialysis chair may lead to changes in balance, lack of sensory stimulation, and, over time, muscle atrophy. In the general population, elderly individuals who report having been restricted to bed for short periods (more than half a day in the past month) are more prone to falls, disability, hospitalization, and mortality.[61] It is difficult to study the impact of a 4-hour dialysis session on hard outcomes such as hospitalization or falls, but one can hypothesize that there are mechanical consequences from sitting or lying for treatment sessions in a proportion of patients, at least. There are some data suggesting that a proportion of patients have a decrease in their postural stability in the immediate postdialysis period. In a small single-center study, 14 patients aged 60 years or older agreed to undergo balance and mobility

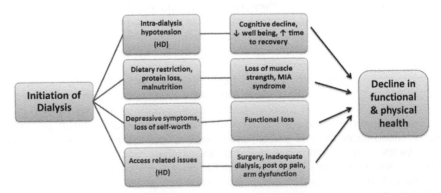

Fig. 3. Effect of dialysis initiation on a variety of health issues. Collectively these may accentuate worsening of geriatric morbidity. MIA, malnutrition, inflammation, and atherosclerosis.

testing immediately before and after a dialysis treatment. The results, though highly variable from patient to patient, showed a decrease in postural stability in the results of tests done after dialysis in several patients.[62] Clinical data also suggest that dialysis itself may affect the risk of falls. In a single-center study of community-dwelling seniors, falls were more common on dialysis days (1.45 vs 1.34 falls per person on dialysis days and nondialysis days, respectively) and, if seen on dialysis days, 3-fold more common after dialysis than before dialysis.[63] Similar findings have been reported by others.[64,65]

Cognitive impairment is underrecognized in the dialysis population.[66–70] Although large epidemiologic studies of HD patients suggest that 15% to 25% of patients have cognitive impairment, intensive studies, specifically designed to detect cognitive change, suggest the burden to be significantly higher.[67] In studies of patients of all ages, more than 77% of prevalent HD patients and 67% of prevalent PD patients showed moderate to severe cognitive impairment on formal testing.[69] Longitudinal studies suggest that this starts early in the course of CKD, and progresses at a more rapid rate than expected from non-CKD populations.[68,71–73] Medication and treatment adherence can be affected by cognitive impairment, particularly as many physicians make on-the-spot changes to medications and treatments during in-centre dialysis rounds. Few interventions seem to be effective in preventing or reducing cognitive impairment in this population. Trials have not conclusively shown any benefits from statin therapy or erythrocyte-stimulating agents, and although early studies suggested a potential benefit from increased dialysis dose (but not frequency),[74,75] this has not been borne out in the recent results from the Frequent Hemodialysis Network trials.[67,69,76–81] Recent studies suggest that cognitive function is worst after the first hour of an HD session, and that poor perfusion of the brain coupled with underlying vascular changes likely influence much of the changes seen.[70,82–85]

SPECIFIC SOLUTIONS FOR GERIATRIC ESRD PATIENTS

As already noted, both cross-sectional and longitudinal studies suggest that patients, initiated on either PD or HD, have an increasing burden of functional disability particularly around the time of dialysis initiation.[16,53,54] As the population ages, more individuals have barriers to self-care. Among these barriers are the high prevalence of physical and cognitive impairments.[55,67,69,86] In the geriatric literature it is well known that poor functional status has an impact on the overall health of the individual, and results in an increased need for long-term care, greater use of formal and informal home services, and an increased burden on caregivers and health care resources.[87–90] Earlier identification of these barriers may lead to prevention of these outcomes through increased support, particularly after acute hospitalization and/or after illness.

The American Society of Nephrology, Geriatric Advisory Group advocates that all elderly CKD patients undergo regular comprehensive geriatric assessment (CGA).[91] The CGA incorporates formal and informal evaluation of the home environment and social support structure; medical history, including treatment targets; functional history; and an assessment of personal values and lifestyle preferences. This information is then coupled with a full assessment of strength, sensory function, balance, cognition, depression, nutrition, and communication skills, and is used to identify potential areas of concern.[92] Multidisciplinary teams can use the results of the assessment to coordinate care in a way that minimizes the functional and/or cognitive stress on elderly individuals, and helps to keep them in their home setting with less burden placed on caregivers.[59]

Geriatric rehabilitation is a therapeutic strategy that may help patients who have experienced a recent decline in functional independence or cognitive function.[59] Rehabilitation can be offered in many forms, some of which include short-stay and slow-stream inpatient programs, outpatient programs, or consultation in the patient's home. Specific interventions used may include therapeutic exercises, fall-prevention plans, education on ways to conserve energy during activity, and recommendation of assistive devices.[59] In the inpatient geriatric rehabilitation setting, initial results appear good among dialysis patients, with more than 70% of patients meeting functional goals and showing improvements.[93,94] Other models of geriatric rehabilitation (including outpatient rehabilitation, community rehabilitation, tele-rehabilitation, and falls prevention programs) have not been well studied in the elderly renal population, but have been shown to benefit other clinical geriatric populations and thus warrant further investigation among the CKD population. Consultation with various allied health specialists (including physiotherapists, occupational therapists, speech-language pathologists, social workers, psychologists, pharmacists, dieticians, and recreation therapists), particularly at transitionary stages of the patient's disease trajectory, is an important component of care for the elderly patient, which can increase the patient's chances of coping with whatever treatment option is pursued.

SUMMARY

The use of dialysis for the treatment of older patients with ESRD is increasing. Although many patients experience increased morbidity and mortality in the early postdialysis period, the use of dialysis therapy should not be considered futile in all cases. Strategies to help patients and their families face the early hurdles to well-being, such as rehabilitation or multidisciplinary support, are being developed. Patients and families should be educated around the role of dialysis withholding or withdrawal, and perhaps in some cases to place less emphasis on immediate access creation or fluid and electrolyte control. The use of treatments such as rehabilitation that improves functional well-being require further testing, but may offer solutions that will help to increase the number of healthy seniors on dialysis in the future.

REFERENCES

1. Report UD. Table B.7 Prevalence of reported ESRD by primary diagnosis by age (page 224). 2012 [cited 2013 28 February]. Available at: http://www.usrds.org/2012/slides/indiv/v2index.html#. Accessed February 28, 2013.
2. Farrington K, Rao R, Gilg J, et al. New adult patients starting renal replacement therapy in the UK in 2005 (chapter 3). Nephrol Dial Transplant 2007;22(Suppl 7):vii11–29.
3. Report UD. Table B.1 Point prevalent counts of reported ESRD patients (page 219). 2012 [cited 2013 28 February]. Available at: http://www.usrds.org/2012/slides/indiv/v2index.html#. Accessed February 28, 2013.
4. Canaud B, Tong L, Tentori F, et al. Clinical practices and outcomes in elderly hemodialysis patients: results from the Dialysis Outcomes and Practice Patterns Study (DOPPS). Clin J Am Soc Nephrol 2011;6(7):1651–62.
5. O'Hare AM, Rodriguez RA, Hailpern SM, et al. Regional variation in health care intensity and treatment practices for end-stage renal disease in older adults. JAMA 2010;304(2):180–6.
6. Dor A, Pauly MV, Eichleay MA, et al. End-stage renal disease and economic incentives: the International Study of Health Care Organization and Financing (ISHCOF). Int J Health Care Finance Econ 2007;7(2–3):73–111.

7. Hemmelgarn BR, James MT, Manns BJ, et al. Rates of treated and untreated kidney failure in older vs younger adults. JAMA 2012;307(23):2507–15.
8. Hsu CY, Vittinghoff E, Lin F, et al. The incidence of end-stage renal disease is increasing faster than the prevalence of chronic renal insufficiency. Ann Intern Med 2004;141(2):95–101.
9. Wald R, Quinn RR, Luo J, et al. Chronic dialysis and death among survivors of acute kidney injury requiring dialysis. JAMA 2009;302(11):1179–85.
10. Lo LJ, Go AS, Chertow GM, et al. Dialysis-requiring acute renal failure increases the risk of progressive chronic kidney disease. Kidney Int 2009;76(8):893–9.
11. Gilbertson DT, Liu J, Xue JL, et al. Projecting the number of patients with end-stage renal disease in the United States to the year 2015. J Am Soc Nephrol 2005;16(12):3736–41.
12. Carson RC, Juszczak M, Davenport A, et al. Is maximal conservative management an equivalent treatment option to dialysis for eldelry patients with significant comorbid disease. Clin J Am Soc Nephrol 2009;4:1611–9.
13. Kurella M, Covinsky KE, Collins AJ, et al. Octogenarians and nonagenarians starting dialysis in the United States. Ann Intern Med 2007;146(3):177–83.
14. Jassal SV, Trpeski L, Zhu N, et al. Changes in survival among elderly patients initiating dialysis from 1990 to 1999. CMAJ 2007;177(9):1033–8.
15. Tamura MK. Incidence, management, and outcomes of end-stage renal disease in the elderly. Curr Opin Nephrol Hypertens 2009;18(3):252–7.
16. Kurella Tamura M, Covinsky KE, Chertow GM, et al. Functional status of elderly adults before and after initiation of dialysis. N Engl J Med 2009;361(16):1539–47.
17. Soucie JM, McClellan WM. Early death in dialysis patients: risk factors and impact on incidence and mortality rates. J Am Soc Nephrol 1996;7(10):2169–75.
18. Bradbury BD, Fissell RB, Albert JM, et al. Predictors of early mortality among incident US hemodialysis patients in the Dialysis Outcomes and Practice Patterns Study (DOPPS). Clin J Am Soc Nephrol 2007;2(1):89–99.
19. McQuillan R, Trpeski L, Fenton S, et al. Modifiable risk factors for early mortality on hemodialysis. Int J Nephrol 2012;2012:435736.
20. Chandna SM, Schulz J, Lawrence C, et al. Is there a rationale for rationing chronic dialysis? A hospital based cohort study of factors affecting survival and morbidity. BMJ 1999;318(7178):217–23.
21. Postorino M, Marino C, Tripepi G, et al. Prognostic value of the New York Heart Association classification in end-stage renal disease. Nephrol Dial Transplant 2007;22(5):1377–82.
22. Rakowski DA, Caillard S, Agodoa LY, et al. Dementia as a predictor of mortality in dialysis patients. Clin J Am Soc Nephrol 2006;1(5):1000–5.
23. Plantinga LC, Fink NE, Levin NW, et al. Early, intermediate, and long-term risk factors for mortality in incident dialysis patients: the Choices for Healthy Outcomes in Caring for ESRD (CHOICE) Study. Am J Kidney Dis 2007;49(6):831–40.
24. O'Hare A, Johansen K. Lower-extremity peripheral arterial disease among patients with end-stage renal disease. J Am Soc Nephrol 2001;12(12):2838–47.
25. Ishii H, Kumada Y, Takahashi H, et al. Impact of diabetes and glycaemic control on peripheral artery disease in Japanese patients with end-stage renal disease: long-term follow-up study from the beginning of haemodialysis. Diabetologia 2012;55(5):1304–9.
26. Morton RL, Snelling P, Webster AC, et al. Dialysis modality preference of patients with CKD and family caregivers: a discrete-choice study. Am J Kidney Dis 2012;60(1):102–11.

27. Kutner NG. Promoting functioning and well being in older CKD patients. Int Urol Nephrol 2008;40:1151–8.
28. Kutner NG, Jassal SV. Quality of life and rehabilitation of elderly dialysis patients. Semin Dial 2002;15(2):107–12.
29. Jassal SV, Watson D. Dialysis in late life: benefit or burden. Clin J Am Soc Nephrol 2009;12:2008–12.
30. O'Hare AM, Bertenthal D, Walter LC, et al. When to refer patients with chronic kidney disease for vascular access surgery: should age be a consideration? Kidney Int 2007;71(6):555–61.
31. Vachharajani TJ, Moossavi S, Jordan JR, et al. Re-evaluating the Fistula First Initiative in octogenarians on hemodialysis. Clin J Am Soc Nephrol 2011;6(7):1663–7.
32. Moist LM, Lok CE, Vachharajani TJ, et al. Optimal hemodialysis vascular access in the elderly patient. Semin Dial 2012;25(6):640–8.
33. ASN Geriatric Nephrology Curriculum. [cited 2013 28 February]. Available at: http://www.asn-online.org/education_and_meetings/distancelearning/curricula/geriatrics/. Accessed February 28, 2013.
34. Ethier J, Mendelssohn DC, Elder SJ, et al. Vascular access use and outcomes: an International Perspective from the Dialysis Outcomes and Practice Patterns Study. Nephrol Dial Transplant 2008;23(10):3219–26.
35. Pisoni RL, Arrington CJ, Albert JM, et al. Facility hemodialysis vascular access use and mortality in countries participating in DOPPS: an instrumental variable analysis. Am J Kidney Dis 2009;53(3):475–91.
36. Lok CE, Allon M, Moist L, et al. Risk equation determining unsuccessful cannulation events and failure to maturation in arteriovenous fistulas (REDUCE FTM I). J Am Soc Nephrol 2006;17(11):3204–12.
37. Lok CE, Oliver MJ, Su J, et al. Arteriovenous fistula outcomes in the era of the elderly dialysis population. Kidney Int 2005;67(6):2462–9.
38. Jassal SV, Watson D. Offering peritoneal dialysis to the older patient: medical progress or waste of time? Semin Nephrol 2011;31(2):225–34.
39. Castrale C, Evans D, Verger C, et al. Peritoneal dialysis in elderly patients: report from the French Peritoneal Dialysis Registry (RDPLF). Nephrol Dial Transplant 2010;25(1):255–62.
40. Lamping DL, Constantinovici N, Roderick P, et al. Clinical outcomes, quality of life, and costs in the North Thames Dialysis Study of elderly people on dialysis: a prospective cohort study. Lancet 2000;356(9241):1543–50.
41. Brown EA, Johansson L, Farrington K, et al. Broadening Options for Long-term Dialysis in the Elderly (BOLDE): differences in quality of life on peritoneal dialysis compared to haemodialysis for older patients. Nephrol Dial Transplant 2010;25(11):3755–63.
42. Oliver MJ, Garg AX, Blake PG, et al. Impact of contraindications, barriers to self-care and support on incident peritoneal dialysis utilization. Nephrol Dial Transplant 2010;25(8):2737–44.
43. Oliver MJ, Quinn RR, Richardson EP, et al. Home care assistance and the utilization of peritoneal dialysis. Kidney Int 2007;71(7):673–8.
44. Lobbedez T, Verger C, Ryckelynck JP, et al. Is assisted peritoneal dialysis associated with technique survival when competing events are considered? Clin J Am Soc Nephrol 2012;7(4):612–8.
45. Povlsen JV, Ivarsen P. Assisted peritoneal dialysis. Adv Chronic Kidney Dis 2007;14(3):279–83.

46. Povlsen JV, Ivarsen P. Assisted automated peritoneal dialysis (AAPD) for the functionally dependent and elderly patient. Perit Dial Int 2005;25(Suppl 3):S60–3.

47. Boudville N, Kemp A, Clayton P, et al. Recent peritonitis associates with mortality among patients treated with peritoneal dialysis. J Am Soc Nephrol 2012;23(8):1398–405.

48. van Esch S, Krediet RT, Struijk DG. Prognostic factors for peritonitis outcome. Contrib Nephrol 2012;178:264–70.

49. Quintanar Lartundo JA, Palomar R, Dominguez-Diez A, et al. Microbiological profile of peritoneal dialysis peritonitis and predictors of hospitalization. Adv Perit Dial 2011;27:38–42.

50. Okayama M, Inoue T, Nodaira Y, et al. Aging is an important risk factor for peritoneal dialysis-associated peritonitis. Adv Perit Dial 2012;28:50–4.

51. Lim WH, Dogra GK, McDonald SP, et al. Compared with younger peritoneal dialysis patients, elderly patients have similar peritonitis-free survival and lower risk of technique failure, but higher risk of peritonitis-related mortality. Perit Dial Int 2011;31(6):663–71.

52. Nessim SJ, Bargman JM, Austin PC, et al. Impact of age on peritonitis risk in peritoneal dialysis patients: an era effect. Clin J Am Soc Nephrol 2009;4(1):135–41.

53. Jassal SV, Chiu E, Hladunewich M. Loss of independence in patients starting dialysis at 80 years of age or older [letter]. N Engl J Med 2009;361(16):1612–3.

54. Thakar CV, Quate-Operacz M, Leonard AC, et al. Outcomes of hemodialysis patients in a long-term care hospital setting: a single-center study. Am J Kidney Dis 2010;55(2):300–6.

55. Cook WL, Jassal SV. Functional dependencies among the elderly on hemodialysis. Kidney Int 2008;73(11):1289–95.

56. Johansen KL, Chertow GM, Jin C, et al. Significance of frailty among dialysis patients. J Am Soc Nephrol 2007;18(11):2960–7.

57. Jaber BL, Lee Y, Collins AJ, et al. Effect of daily hemodialysis on depressive symptoms and postdialysis recovery time: interim report from the FREEDOM (Following Rehabilitation, Economics and Everyday-Dialysis Outcome Measurements) Study. Am J Kidney Dis 2010;56(3):531–9.

58. Lindsay RM, Heidenheim PA, Nesrallah G, et al. Minutes to recovery after a hemodialysis session: a simple health-related quality of life question that is reliable, valid, and sensitive to change. Clin J Am Soc Nephrol 2006;1(5):952–9.

59. Farragher J, Jassal SV. Rehabilitation of the geriatric dialysis patient. Semin Dial 2012;25(6):649–56.

60. Delgado C, Johansen KL. Barriers to exercise participation among dialysis patients. Nephrol Dial Transplant 2012;27(3):1152–7.

61. Gill TM, Allore HG, Gahbauer EA, et al. Change in disability after hospitalization or restricted activity in older persons. JAMA 2010;304(17):1919–28.

62. Sims RJ, Taylor R, Masud T, et al. The effect of a single haemodialysis session on functional mobility in older adults: a pilot study. Int Urol Nephrol 2007;39(4):1287–93.

63. Cook WL, Tomlinson G, Donaldson M, et al. Falls and fall-related injuries in older dialysis patients. Clin J Am Soc Nephrol 2006;1(6):1197–204.

64. Abdel-Rahman EM, Turgut F, Turkmen K, et al. Falls in elderly hemodialysis patients. QJM 2011;104(10):829–38.

65. Desmet C, Beguin C, Swine C, et al. Falls in hemodialysis patients: prospective study of incidence, risk factors, and complications. Am J Kidney Dis 2005;45(1):148–53.

66. Folstein MF, Folstein SE, McHugh PR. "Mini-mental state". A practical method for grading the cognitive state of patients for the clinician. J Psychiatr Res 1975; 12(3):189–98.

67. Murray AM. Cognitive impairment in hemodialysis patients is common. Neurology 2006;67(2):216–23.

68. McQuillan R, Jassal SV. Neuropsychiatric complications of chronic kidney disease [review]. Nat Rev Nephrol 2010;6(8):471–9.

69. Kalirao P, Pederson S, Foley RN, et al. Cognitive impairment in peritoneal dialysis patients. Am J Kidney Dis 2011;57(4):612–20.

70. Sarnak MJ, Tighiouart H, Scott TM, et al. Frequency of and risk factors for poor cognitive performance in hemodialysis patients. Neurology 2013;80(5): 471–80.

71. Kurella M. Chronic kidney disease and cognitive impairment in the elderly: the health, aging, and body composition study. J Am Soc Nephrol 2005;16(7): 2127–33.

72. Yaffe K, Ackerson L, Tamura MK, et al. Chronic kidney disease and cognitive function in older adults: findings from the chronic renal insufficiency cohort cognitive study. J Am Geriatr Soc 2010;58(2):338–45.

73. Kurella Tamura M, Xie D, Yaffe K, et al. Vascular risk factors and cognitive impairment in chronic kidney disease: the Chronic Renal Insufficiency Cohort (CRIC) study. Clin J Am Soc Nephrol 2011;6(2):248–56.

74. Jassal SV, Devins GM, Chan CT, et al. Improvements in cognition in patients converting from thrice weekly hemodialysis to nocturnal hemodialysis: a longitudinal pilot study. Kidney Int 2006;70(5):956–62.

75. Vos PF, Zilch O, Jennekens-Schinkel A, et al. Effect of short daily home haemodialysis on quality of life, cognitive functioning and the electroencephalogram. Nephrol Dial Transplant 2006;21(9):2529–35.

76. Chertow GM, Levin NW, Beck GJ, et al. In-center hemodialysis six times per week versus three times per week. N Engl J Med 2010;363(24):2287–300.

77. Kurella Tamura M, Unruh ML, Nissenson AR, et al. Effect of more frequent hemodialysis on cognitive function in the frequent hemodialysis network trials. Am J Kidney Dis 2013;61(2):228–37.

78. Kurella Tamura M, Yaffe K. Dementia and cognitive impairment in ESRD: diagnostic and therapeutic strategies. Kidney Int 2011;79(1):14–22.

79. Kurella Tamura M, Larive B, Unruh ML, et al. Prevalence and correlates of cognitive impairment in hemodialysis patients: the Frequent Hemodialysis Network trials. Clin J Am Soc Nephrol 2010;5(8):1429–38.

80. Griva K, Stygall J, Hankins M, et al. Cognitive impairment and 7-year mortality in dialysis patients. Am J Kidney Dis 2010;56(4):693–703.

81. Kurella M, Mapes DL, Port FK, et al. Correlates and outcomes of dementia among dialysis patients: the Dialysis Outcomes and Practice Patterns Study. Nephrol Dial Transplant 2006;21(9):2543–8.

82. Drew DA, Bhadelia R, Tighiouart H, et al. Anatomic brain disease in hemodialysis patients: a cross-sectional Study. Am J Kidney Dis 2013;61(2):271–8.

83. Kurella Tamura M, Meyer JB, Saxena AB, et al. Prevalence and significance of stroke symptoms among patients receiving maintenance dialysis. Neurology 2012;79(10):981–7.

84. Harciarek M, Williamson JB, Biedunkiewicz B, et al. Risk factors for selective cognitive decline in dialyzed patients with end-stage renal disease: evidence from verbal fluency analysis. J Int Neuropsychol Soc 2012;18(1): 162–7.

85. Kim CD, Lee HJ, Kim DJ, et al. High prevalence of leukoaraiosis in cerebral magnetic resonance images of patients on peritoneal dialysis. Am J Kidney Dis 2007;50(1):98–107.

86. Lo D, Chiu E, Jassal SV. A prospective pilot study to measure changes in functional status associated with hospitalization in elderly dialysis-dependent patients. Am J Kidney Dis 2008;52(5):956–61.

87. Manton KG, Gu X, Lamb VL. Change in chronic disability from 1982 to 2004/2005 as measured by long-term changes in function and health in the U.S. elderly population. Proc Natl Acad Sci 2006;103(48):18374–9.

88. Carey EC, Covinsky KE, Lui LY, et al. Prediction of mortality in community-living frail elderly people with long-term care needs. J Am Geriatr Soc 2008;56(1): 68–75.

89. Mehta KM, Yaffe K, Brenes GA, et al. Anxiety symptoms and decline in physical function over 5 years in the health, aging and body composition study. J Am Geriatr Soc 2007;55(2):265–70.

90. Covinsky KE, Eng C, Lui LY, et al. The last 2 years of life: functional trajectories of frail older people. J Am Geriatr Soc 2003;51(4):492–8.

91. Rosner M, Abdel-Rahman E, Williams ME. Geriatric nephrology: responding to a growing challenge. Clin J Am Soc Nephrol 2010;5(5):936–42.

92. ASN Geriatric Nephrology: improving dialysis rounds. 2012 [cited 2013]. Available at: http://www.asn-online.org/kidneydisease/geriatrics/rounds/. Accessed 2013.

93. Jassal SV, Chiu E, Li M. Geriatric hemodialysis rehabilitation care. Adv Chronic Kidney Dis 2008;15(2):115–22.

94. Li M, Porter E, Lam R, et al. Quality improvement through the introduction of interdisciplinary geriatric hemodialysis rehabilitation care. Am J Kidney Dis 2007;50(1):90–7.

Decision Making in Elderly Patients with Advanced Kidney Disease

Holly M. Koncicki, MD, MS[a,b,*], Mark A. Swidler, MD[a,b]

KEYWORDS

- Dialysis • Nondialysis medical therapy • Elderly • Chronic kidney disease
- End-stage renal disease • Palliative care

KEY POINTS

- When caring for elderly patients with chronic kidney disease, a thoughtful approach to shared decision making can be accomplished using the 4 topics of shared decision making: medical indications, patient preferences, quality of life, and contextual features.
- Prognosis should be determined based on disease trajectories and the assessment of functional age, and placed in the context of patient preferences, values and goals of care.
- The Renal Physician Association's guidelines provide useful information when recommending dialysis or nondialysis medical therapy. Regardless of the treatment path taken, patient prognosis, preferences, and quality of life should be reevaluated regularly and during sentinel events using an advance-care-planning and family meeting format.
- Integrating geriatric renal palliative care concepts is beneficial in caring for elderly patients with chronic kidney disease by providing symptom management and helping with the difficult decisions and transitions of care that will arise during the clinical course of elderly patients with renal disease.

Learning objectives

1. To review the 4-topic framework and ethical principles involved in shared decision making

2. To describe useful prognostic factors when evaluating elderly patients for dialysis or nondialysis medical therapy

3. To review the role of geriatric renal palliative care in management of advanced kidney disease

---

Disclosures: None.
Conflict of Interest: None.
[a] Nephrology, Department of Medicine, Icahn School of Medicine at Mount Sinai, One Gustave L. Levy Place, Box 1243, New York, NY 10029, USA; [b] Department of Geriatrics and Palliative Medicine, Icahn School of Medicine at Mount Sinai, One Gustave L. Levy Place, Box 1070, New York, NY 10029, USA
* Corresponding author.
E-mail address: holly.koncicki@mssm.edu

Clin Geriatr Med 29 (2013) 641–655
http://dx.doi.org/10.1016/j.cger.2013.05.004
0749-0690/13/$ – see front matter © 2013 Elsevier Inc. All rights reserved.

INTRODUCTION

The decisions about whether and when to initiate dialysis can be difficult and imprecise and are traditionally guided by criteria, such as renal function (measured by glomerular filtration rate [GFR]) and uremic symptoms. For elderly patients with renal disease facing these decisions, an added layer of complexity is present because the assessment of functional status, comorbidities, and geriatric syndromes is required, all of which predict adverse outcomes.[1–7] In addition, renal replacement therapy is associated with loss of independence, functional decline, increased morbidity, and substantial mortality in elderly patients.[8–10] Because the fastest-growing group of patients initiating dialysis is older than 75 years, geriatricians will be more involved in decisions regarding the appropriate treatment of end-stage renal disease (ESRD).[11]

Chronic kidney disease (CKD) is associated with an increased prevalence of geriatric syndromes, including frailty, functional disability, and cognitive impairment.[2,3,12,13] Symptoms associated with these syndromes, particularly frailty, may mimic uremic manifestations and precipitate the initiation of dialysis with the hope of improving functional status.[14] A recent study showed that frail elderly patients with renal disease, defined by the Fried Frailty Screening Tool,[15] were more often initiated on dialysis at a higher GFR and demonstrated increased rates of hospitalizations and increased mortality. These outcomes were independently associated with frailty, suggesting that frail patients are being started on dialysis earlier and without benefit.[14]

Several studies have demonstrated adverse effects on functional status after the initiation of dialysis in elderly patients.[8,9,14] One study showed that in the 6 months following dialysis initiation in a group of patients older than 80 years living independently, 30% experienced functional decline and loss of independence requiring increased caregiver support or transfer to a nursing home.[8] Another study of nursing home patients who started dialysis found that 61% of residents either died or had a decline in functional status at 3 months, which increased to 87% at 12 months.[9] Factors independently associated with a lower odds ratio of maintaining predialysis functional status included older age, white race, cerebrovascular disease, dementia, hypoalbuminemia less than 3.5 g/dL, and hospitalization at the time of dialysis initiation. Additional reasons for functional decline in this nursing home dialysis population included a high prevalence of disability; poor baseline functional status before the start of dialysis; and psychosocial burdens, like decreased time for physical activity, missed social experiences, such as mealtimes, and increased symptoms.[9]

GUIDELINES FOR MEDICAL DECISION MAKING

Both ESRD and the dialysis trajectory have characteristics of a chronic disease model, including decreased life expectancy compared with age-matched populations, progressive disability, repeated hospitalizations, increased comorbidities, high symptom burden, and caregiver stress.[16] Patients rely on their medical team for health information, emotional support, and decision-making guidance. More than 80% of patients with CKD or ESRD think it is important to be aware of all treatment options, including withdrawing from dialysis, advance care planning (ACP), and symptom management; however, information about these choices is not readily available.[17] One study showed that 61% of patients regretted their decision to start dialysis, which was driven by their physician's or family's preference.[17] This finding illustrates the importance of a shared decision in which the physician informs patients of the risks and benefits while also exploring patient preferences and values when discussing the 2 ESRD treatment options of dialysis or nondialysis medical therapy (NDMT). Based on this discussion, the physician should make a recommendation regarding treatment but should be prepared that disagreements may occur.[18]

Shared decision making can be approached by considering a 4-topic framework that includes medical indications, patient preferences, quality of life (QOL), and contextual features.[18,19] Medical indications for dialysis or NDMT assess whether patients are better candidates for one modality or the other from a purely medical standpoint. This process involves the evaluation of the patients' comorbid conditions, overall prognosis, and disease trajectory and then inclusion of this information in the discussion about treatment options with patients or their health care decision maker.[18]

To formulate a prognosis in elderly patients with renal disease, functional age should be estimated by performing a geriatric assessment that includes functional status, frailty and cognitive testing, and comorbidity scores.[16] Although not yet validated in the CKD/ESRD population, functional age is commonly used in geriatric oncology for decision making regarding cancer treatment.[20–22] Patients can be placed in 1 of 3 functional age categories as outlined in **Table 1**.[16,20–24] Based on these categories, a medical recommendation might be made for dialysis in healthy patients and NDMT or a time-limited trial of dialysis in elderly, frail patients with renal disease.

Discussing the benefits and burdens of ESRD treatment options reflect underlying ethical principles of beneficence and nonmaleficence.[18] Burdens associated with dialysis include surgery for dialysis access, duration of dialysis therapy (indefinite if not a transplant candidate), individual time session (3–4 hours), transportation issues, and hospitalizations for various medical events. Although NDMT is generally associated with shortened survival versus dialysis, benefits include improved QOL, less hospitalizations, and more deaths at home.[6,25–27] In elderly patients with renal disease with high comorbidity scores or ischemic heart disease, survival may be similar in both NDMT and dialysis.[6] Regardless of the therapy choice, renal palliative care input to help update ACP and address the physical symptoms and the psychological, spiritual, and cultural needs of patients and families is recommended.[28,29]

Patient preferences are reflected in the informed consent process, which explores personal values, beliefs, and burdens versus benefits and embodies the ethical principle of autonomy.[18] If the patient does not have decision-making capacity, a health care proxy or surrogate should be included in these discussions.

The QOL topic examines big-picture goals aiming for those that are realistic and matches them to the appropriate treatments that can achieve them.[18] It is reflective of the ethical principles of autonomy and beneficence. Starter questions to explore QOL might include the following: What makes your life worth living? Has anyone in your family or among your friends ever been on dialysis? What was it like for them? What was it like for you to see them getting this treatment?

Lastly, contextual features reflect the ethical principle of justice and explore other patient aspects, such as social, financial, institutional, psychological, and spiritual issues that may affect decision making.[18] Resolving conflict between family members or between family and the health teams and arriving at a consensus regarding the medical decision is an important component of this topic.

Exploring the aforementioned topics will help make a recommendation that best suits each patient. The Renal Physicians Association (RPA) has developed evidence-based guidelines for physicians and patients regarding initiation or withdrawal of dialysis.[30] The guidelines recommend that physicians share prognosis with patients, including a prediction of their performance on dialysis, and involve palliative care to help with symptom management and ACP.[30] A time-limited trial with clear predefined targets like improvement in cognition or functional status or an acceptable QOL can be

Table 1
Functional age

Functional Age	Clinical Description		Recommendations for Renal Replacement Therapy
Healthy/usual or fit	• Few hospitalizations • Good QOL	• KPS ≥80 • Independent in ADLs and iADLs • Low comorbidity score (CCI ≤4) • No geriatric syndromes (dementia, frailty, functional disability, depression, malnutrition, falls) • Negative physical frailty testing[a] • Answer *yes* to the surprise question	• Optimal for dialysis or transplant
Vulnerable or intermediate	• Increasing hospitalizations	• KPS 50–80 • Dependent in one ADL and iADLs • Comorbidity score (CCI 5–7), REIN clinical score <9 • 1–2 geriatric syndromes • Prefrail (1–2 criteria) to + frailty testing[a] • Unclear answer to surprise question: I don't know	• Typical dialysis patient • Assessment of and intervention on geriatric issues to optimize factors that may adversely affect outcomes
Frail	• Susceptible to poor outcomes • High risk of hospitalizations • Nursing home patients with notable disability	KPS <50 • Dependent in >2 ADLs and iADLS • Significant symptom burden • Answer *no* to the surprise question • High comorbidity score (CCI ≥8), REIN score ≥9 • >2 geriatric syndromes • Physical frailty • Cognitive dysfunction • Inability to transfer	• Suboptimal dialysis candidate • Recommend NDMT or time-limited trial of dialysis

Karnofsky Performance Score: 100: normal, no complaints, no evidence of disease; 80: normal activity with effort, some symptoms or signs of disease; 50: requires considerable assistance and frequent medical care.

Abbreviations: ADL, activities of daily living; CCI,[36] Charlson Comorbidity Index (see text); iADL, instrumental activities of daily living; KPS, Karnofsky Performance Scale; REIN score,[5] Renal Epidemiology and Information Network Prognosis score (see text).

[a] Physical frailty[15] means 3 or more of the following criteria: unintentional weight loss of more than 10 lb in last year, self-reported exhaustion, weakness (grip strength), slow walking speed, low physical activity.

Data from Swidler M. Chapter 37, Dialysis decisions in the elderly patient with advanced CKD and the role of nondialytictherapy. In: Oreopoulos D, Wiggins J, editors. American Society of Nephrology Geriatric Nephrology Curriculum. Washington, DC: American Society of Nephrology; 2009. http://www.asn-online.org/education/distancelearning/curricula/geriatrics/Chapter37.pdf. Accessed February 3, 2013.

offered if the prognosis is unclear or a decision regarding dialysis cannot be made. ACP and reevaluation of the prognosis either yearly or following a sentinel event or change in clinical status is also recommended. Forgoing (withholding or withdrawing) dialysis can be considered if[30]

- Requested voluntarily by a patient who has decision-making capacity and has been fully informed of risks and benefits
- A patient without decision-making capacity has previous oral or written advance directives describing a decision to forgo dialysis or at the request of the legal health care proxy or surrogate
- A patient has irreversible and profound neurologic impairment without signs of thought, sensation, purposeful behavior, and awareness
- A patient has a nonrenal terminal illness
- Dialysis cannot be safely provided because of hemodynamic instability or underlying conditions with significant behavioral issues.

PROGNOSTICATION AND DISEASE TRAJECTORIES

Up to 90% of patients with CKD and ESRD want information regarding prognosis, but actual discussions occur infrequently.[17] In one study, less than 20% of patients surveyed expected their health to deteriorate over the next 12 months, although the age-based 3-year life expectancy was only 50%.[17] Sharing prognoses and developing realistic expectations with patients and families can also be improved by using disease trajectories that outline the temporal course of a chronic disease. This practice allows for the opportunity to appropriately recommend palliative care and, in the case of ESRD, explore NDMT as an acceptable treatment option for certain subgroups of elderly patients with renal disease.

Chronic medical conditions generally follow 1 of 3 disease trajectories, which have been validated in patients older than 65 years (**Fig. 1**).[31,32] One trajectory, commonly seen in cancer (terminal illness), terminates in an abrupt, surprise death either without preceding functional decline or following a short period of deterioration over weeks to months.[33] A second trajectory characterizes noncancer progressive chronic conditions, such as end-stage chronic obstructive pulmonary disease (COPD), advanced congestive heart failure (CHF), and ESRD on dialysis. This trajectory spans months to years, with acute intermittent episodes of decline correlating with hospitalizations or sentinel events with a failure to return to the previous functional status.[33] Examples of sentinel events in patients undergoing dialysis that often require hospitalization include infections, dialysis access malfunction, limb amputations, and cardiac events. Although patients may survive many acute deteriorations, any one episode can result in death.[33] A third trajectory, commonly seen in frailty or dementia, has a prolonged phase of decreasing functional status and dwindling.[33]

A fourth trajectory was recently described in advanced CKD managed by NDMT.[33–35] A longitudinal cohort study of elderly patients with CKD stage 5, defined as an estimated GFR less than 15 mL/min, managed with NDMT assessed functional status using the Karnofsky Performance Scale (KPS). Functional status remained stable for long periods of time but could change quickly, often with a sharp decline in the 1 to 2 months before death.[35] Because CKD is commonly associated with multiple comorbidities, multiple disease trajectories can be superimposed on each other, which further complicates predicting the clinical course and prognosis and reinforces the value of palliative care input.[34]

Numerous studies have sought to identify prognostic factors regarding patient performance on dialysis.[1–5,7,10,13,36–40] The RPA's guidelines recommend that NDMT

Profiles of Older Medicare Decedents

Proposed Trajectories of Dying

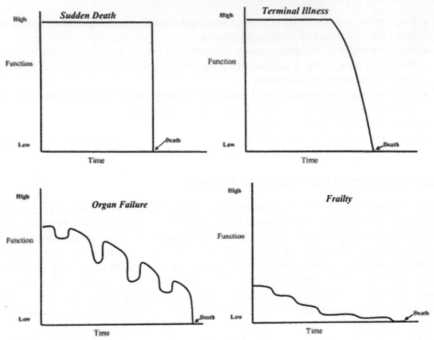

Fig. 1. Trajectories of chronic disease. (*Reprinted from* Lunney JR, Lynn J, Hogan C. Profiles of older Medicare decedents. J Am Geriatr Soc 2002;50:1108–12; with permission from John Wiley and Sons.)

should be considered in patients with CKD stage 5 who are older than 75 years and have 2 of the following poor prognostic indicators[30]:

- Impaired functional status (KPS <40; disabled requiring special care and assistance)
- Severe malnutrition (serum albumin <2 g/dL)
- High comorbidity score (Charlson Comorbidity Index ≥8)
- A positive response to the surprise question (ie, "No, I would be surprised if this patient died within the next year.") (see later discussion)

Age is an important prognostic marker with several studies showing decreased survival in elderly patients starting dialysis compared with a younger population (**Table 2**).[4,10,39,41] This decreased survival may be partly due to initiation of dialysis under suboptimal conditions. When compared with younger (aged 50–60 years) patients, elderly (aged >75 years) patients undergoing new-start dialysis show a trend toward later referral to nephrologists, greater likelihood of hemodialysis compared with peritoneal dialysis, and the use of long-term temporary catheters instead of permanent vascular access.[39]

Similar to the general geriatric population, the presence of falls, cognitive impairment, and frailty are also associated with an increased risk of mortality in elderly

Table 2
Mortality after dialysis initiation

Age (y)	1-y Mortality (%)	Median Survival After Initiation of Dialysis (mo)	Average Life Expectancy in General Population (mo)
70–74	20	24.9	176
75–79	31		138
80–84	46	15.6	105
85–89		11.6	78
>90	46	8.4	57

Data from Refs.[4,10,39,41]

patients with advancing CKD and should be assessed and included in the prognosis evaluation when recommending treatment modality.[1–5,13,37,38]

Frailty is common in the CKD and dialysis populations.[1,2,38] The prevalence of frailty and disability is 2 times higher (15%) in patients with CKD who are older than 65 years compared with age-matched patients (6%) with normal renal function.[2] CKD was also shown to be a risk factor for developing frailty in a prospective study that found an association between CKD and incident functional impairment that was independent of comorbidity, body composition, strength testing, and physical performance in previously well-functioning elderly patients.[3] In addition, frail patients with CKD are 2.5 times more likely to die or initiate dialysis than their nonfrail counterparts.[38]

In the Dialysis Morbidity and Mortality Wave 2 Study, a cohort of 2275 adult patients undergoing dialysis, the prevalence of frailty was 67.7% and increased with age, with 44% of patients younger than 40 years, 66.4% of patients between 50 and 60 years old, and 78% of patients older than 80 years demonstrating frailty.[1] Mortality was also increased 2.25 times in the frail patients undergoing dialysis.[1] Individual components of frailty, including nonambulatory status and the inability to transfer, are also markers of increased mortality following the initiation of dialysis.[4,5]

Comorbidities are important prognostic markers in patients with advanced CKD and in those receiving dialysis. In a study of patients older than 80 years starting dialysis, the risk of death was 31% in patients with 2 to 3 comorbid conditions and 68% in those with 4 or more comorbid conditions compared with those with 0 to 1 comorbid conditions (comorbid conditions were anemia, CHF, underweight, low albumin, nonambulatory status, diabetes, ischemic heart disease, COPD, cancer, or cerebrovascular disease).[4]

The Charlson Comorbidity Index (CCI) is a score based on age, with one point for every decade over 40 years, and different weights assigned to different comorbid conditions (**Tables 3** and **4**). The CCI was validated in hemodialysis and peritoneal dialysis patients in predicting hospital admission rates, hospital days, and mortality.[36] Patients with a CCI ≥8 had the highest mortality at 0.49 per patient year.[36]

The surprise question (Would I [the physician] be surprised if this patient died in the next year?) is another validated mortality predictor in patients undergoing dialysis; mortality in the *no* group is 3.5 times higher compared with the *yes* group.[7,40] The surprise question has been adapted into a validated 6-month hemodialysis mortality predictor available online (http://touchcalc.com/calculators/sq) that also includes older age, dementia, peripheral vascular disease, and decreased albumin.[7]

Finally, a validated scoring system (Renal Epidemiology and Information Network Prognosis [REIN] score) for 6-month mortality based on 9 variables given different

Table 3 CCI	
Score	Condition
1	Coronary artery disease
	CHF
	Peripheral vascular disease
	Dementia
	Chronic pulmonary disease
	Connective tissue disorder
	Peptic ulcer disease
	Mild liver disease
2	Hemiplegia
	Moderate or severe renal disease
	Diabetes with end-organ damage
	Any tumor, leukemia, lymphoma
3	Moderate or severe liver disease
6	Metastatic solid tumor
	AIDS

An additional 1 point added for every 10 years more than 40 years of age.

weights for patients undergoing dialysis who are older than 75 years is summarized in **Tables 5** and **6**.[5]

NDMT: WHO IS IT FOR?

After discussing prognostic factors and disease trajectories, formulating the patients' functional age and reviewing QOL issues within the framework of the 4-topic decision-making method, NDMT may be an appropriate choice for certain elderly patients with advanced CKD, specifically those who are frail. This decision can be difficult and requires continued support from a multidisciplinary health team with access to increasing home services as the trajectory continues to unfold.

Several studies have identified factors that influence both the physician choice of referral and the patients' decisions to pursue either dialysis or NDMT. Physicians have recommended NDMT for patients with many of the previously discussed poor prognostic markers, like functional disability measured by lower KPS, older age, and higher comorbidity scores.[42] Patients have expressed a preference for dialysis over NDMT if there was an increased life expectancy, flexibility in the time or day of treatment, and subsidized travel. Conversely, NDMT was preferred if patients were

Table 4 CCI score and mortality	
CCI Score	Mortality per Patient-Year (%)
Low ≤3	3
Moderate 4–5	13
High 6–7	27
Very High ≥8	49

Reprinted and Adapted from Beddhu S, Bruns F, Saul M, et al. A simple comorbidity scale predicts clinical outcomes and costs in dialysis patients. Am J Med 2000;108:609–13; with permission from Elsevier.

Table 5	
REIN scoring system	
Points	**Variables**
3	Total dependency for transfers
2	Body mass index <18.5 kg/m^2 CHF stages III to IV Peripheral vascular disease stages III to IV Severe behavioral disorder Unplanned dialysis
1	Diabetes Dysrhythmia Active malignancy

Data from Couchoud C, Labeeuw M, Moranne O, et al. A clinical score to predict 6-month prognosis in elderly patients starting dialysis for end-stage renal disease. Nephrol Dial Transplant 2009;24:1553–61.

older, satisfied with their current QOL, concerned with being a burden on caregivers, and if the treatment was associated with an increased ability to travel and a decreased number of visits to the hospital.[43,44] One study reported that patients were willing to sacrifice 7 months of survival to decrease the number of visits per week to the dialysis unit by one visit and 15 months of survival to increase the ability to travel for leisure.[44]

NDMT: CLINICAL COURSE AND PROGNOSIS

Given the heterogeneous patient populations studied, broad generalizations regarding survival on dialysis compared with NDMT are difficult. For most patients with ESRD, dialysis offers a survival benefit. However, in specific populations and circumstances, this benefit may not be apparent. In one study, patients older than 75 years who chose NDMT had an average survival at 1 and 2 years of 68% and 47% compared with 84% and 76% in a similar population on dialysis.[6] When patients with high comorbidity scores or ischemic heart disease were compared, the survival benefit of dialysis was lost.[6,26,45] A similar study found that patients undergoing dialysis had a median survival of 67 months compared with an NDMT group who survived 21 months with a survival benefit of 46 months; but when controlled for age of more than 75 years and comorbidities, the survival difference decreased to 4 months and was not

Table 6	
Mortality at 6 months	
REIN Score	**Mortality (%)**
0	8
1	10
2	17
3–4	21
5–6	33
7–8	50
>9	70

Data from Couchoud C, Labeeuw M, Moranne O, et al. A clinical score to predict 6-month prognosis in elderly patients starting dialysis for end-stage renal disease. Nephrol Dial Transplant 2009;24:1553–61.

statistically significant.[45] Another study showed that suboptimal dialysis candidates for whom NDMT was recommended but chose dialysis had a nonstatistically significant increase in median survival by 2 months as compared with the NDMT group.[42]

A study[27] of patients older than 70 years with ESRD (GFR <10.8 mL/min) showed a survival advantage in the dialysis versus the NDMT group (37.8 vs 13.9 months) but more hospitalizations (25 days per patient-year vs 16 days). When time lost was considered (hospital admissions, travel and time related to dialysis, and posttreatment fatigue), the hemodialysis group spent 47.5% of the days survived (or 173 days per year) participating in or related to their treatment compared with 4.3% of days (or 16 days per year) in the NDMT group.[27] The NDMT patients were also 4 times more likely to die at home or in hospice.[27]

PALLIATIVE CARE AND HOSPICE

Palliative care is a simultaneous care model for patients with chronic and serious medical conditions that matches medical care to patient goals, is appropriate at any stage of illness alongside targeted therapy, and is not synonymous with end-of-life care.[16,46] As defined by the World Health Organization, its goal is to improve the QOL of patients and their families through prevention and relief of suffering by early identification; assessment and treatment of pain and symptoms; and providing physical, psychosocial, and spiritual support.[25,28]

Geriatric renal palliative care is an example of the simultaneous care model in noncancer chronic illness with an emphasis on geriatric syndromes and guidance with transitions across the health care system for older adults.[24,46] It is appropriate to introduce when the GFR is less than 20 to 30 mL/min (CKD stage 4) and uses a multidisciplinary team approach[26] that continues through the NDMT or dialysis experience and beyond the death of patients, with bereavement support for family and caregivers.[16,28,29] It includes the following components[28,29,47]:

- ACP
- Active treatment of symptoms and geriatric syndromes
- Active medical treatment of renal complications (hypertension, anemia, volume overload, mineral bone disease, and electrolyte abnormalities)
- Patient and family support as disease trajectory progresses
- Hospice referral when appropriate (<6 months estimated survival)

Despite awareness of the symptom burden in patients undergoing dialysis, treatment has been inadequate partly because of poor symptom recognition.[48,49] The mean number of symptoms has ranged from 9.0 in the general dialysis population to 10.5 in patients with high comorbidity scores (CCI ≥8), which is comparable with ambulatory (9.7) and inpatients (11.5) with cancer.[50,51] Patients undergoing NDMT also report a high number of symptoms (6.8–17.0), which can increase in the month before death.[52] Pain is the most common symptom, occurring in 50% to 79% of patients.[48,50] Other significant symptoms include lack of energy, drowsiness, numbness and tingling, dry mouth, poor appetite, dyspnea, edema, difficulty sleeping, and pruritus.[51,52]

ACP is an ongoing interactional process with an emphasis on goals of care and informed decision making (using the family meeting model). Its objectives include optimizing communication between patients, caregivers, and their health care team; decreasing burdens and strengthening relationships; naming a health care proxy (HCP); and specifying wishes for end-of-life care.[25,28] The deaths of patients on dialysis who have advance directives are more reconciled rather than sudden and unexpected,[51,53] yet ACP is not readily used in the ESRD population. In one study of patients on dialysis with high comorbidity scores, the majority (89%) decided on an HCP; but only one-third of the patients completed the paperwork, and a minority discussed end-of-life wishes.[51] ACP discussions are appropriate in the following situations:

- The GFR is less than 20 to 30 mL/min (CKD stage 4 and lower).
- Dialysis versus NDMT decision discussions are being initiated.
- The life expectancy is less than 12 months.
- The prognosis is unclear.
- There is a disease exacerbation or a decline in health or function occurs.

If the answer to the surprise question is *no* during a scheduled prognostic evaluation, the health care team should assess cognition, nutrition, functional status, symptom burden, and patients' QOL to help patients and families recognize the progressive nature of the disease trajectory toward the end-of-life period.[54]

The family meeting, which includes the geriatric renal patient, main decision makers, friends and/or family, and the geriatric renal palliative care team, provides a structured environment for the ACP process. Patients' values and preferences are identified; possible treatment options, including NDMT, are reviewed; and a medical plan is developed that reflects the patients' goals.[25] It is important to assess the patients' and their family's understanding and perception of the medical condition and how much detailed information is desired. Information should be shared, empathy provided, questions addressed, and follow-up established.[25]

The identification of *end of life* is important to prepare patients and families for changes in expectations and care needs, with a referral to hospice when the prognosis is less than 6 months. This period for patients undergoing dialysis may begin with clinical scenarios such as[29] the following:

- Increasing difficultly with dialysis access cannulation, recurrent clotting, revisions, and loss of alternate sites
- Inability to tolerate hemodialysis secondary to hemodynamic instability or peritoneal dialysis failure secondary to loss of ultrafiltration with no other available treatment options
- Increasing number of missed dialysis sessions or shortened treatment time with no reversible factors
- Answering *no* in response to the surprise question
- Infections like catheter-related bacteremia or endocarditis that become recurrent or resistant to treatment
- Increasing symptoms requiring complex management, such as refractory pain, pruritus, or restless legs
- Multiple hospital admissions with complications
- Patients consistently declining medications, oral nutrition, or nursing care with no reversible causes
- Debility manifested by the following:
  - Unintentional weight loss of more than 10% over 3 months
  - Loss of more than 3 activities of daily living over 6 months
  - Decubitus ulcers
  - Increasing bedbound time

Hospice referral is appropriate for any patient who (1) withdraws from dialysis, (2) is treated by NDMT with a prognosis of less than 6 months, or (3) is on dialysis and wishes to continue and has a non-renal terminal disease as the primary diagnosis with a prognosis of less than 6 months.[28]

In the United States, patients with ESRD use hospice services only half as often (20%) when compared with patients with cancer (55%) or heart failure (39%).[54,55] Approximately 42% of patients who withdraw from dialysis enroll in hospice; failure to thrive is a more common hospice enrollment diagnosis than a medical complication.[54] Hospice patients with ESRD are 4 times more likely to die at home than in the hospital, and their per-patient cost of care during the last week of life is significantly less by almost $3000.[54] Therefore, it is important for patients with ESRD to be appropriately identified as hospice candidates to best use their benefits. On average, patients undergoing maintenance dialysis who withdraw from dialysis survive for 10 days.[56]

SUMMARY

When caring for elderly patients with CKD, a thoughtful approach to shared decision making (**Box 1**) can be accomplished using the 4 topics of shared decision making:

Box 1
Approach to decision making in elderly patients with CKD

1. Evaluate the 4 topics of shared decision making[19]:
   a. Medical indications
   b. Patient preferences
   c. QOL
   d. Contextual features
2. Estimate patient prognosis (see text).
   a. Determine functional age of patients.
      i. Healthy/usual or fit
      ii. Vulnerable or intermediate
      iii. Frail
   b. Use disease trajectories to predict clinical course (see text).
3. Discuss recommendations with patients and families.
   a. Develop a treatment plan based on the aforementioned factors in a shared decision with patients and families.
   b. If disagreement exists, or prognosis is unclear, offer a time-limited trial of dialysis with predefined targets.
4. Integrate a geriatric renal palliative care approach at CKD stage 4 to
   a. Continue predialysis care: treatment of anemia, mineral bone disease, volume status, hypertension, hyperlipidemia, and electrolyte abnormalities
   b. Discuss ACP
      i. To aid in communication with patients and caregivers
      ii. To decrease burdens and strengthen relationships
      iii. To name an HCP
      iv. Specify wishes for the end of life
   c. Control symptoms
   d. Assess and treat geriatric syndromes
   e. Provide practical, psychosocial, and spiritual care to patients and families/caregivers

medical indications, patient preferences, QOL, and contextual features. The prognosis should be determined based on disease trajectories (see **Fig. 1**) and the assessment of functional age (see **Table 1**) and placed in the context of patient preferences, values, and goals of care. The RPA's guidelines provide useful information when recommending dialysis or NDMT. Regardless of the treatment path taken, patient prognosis, preferences, and QOL should be reevaluated regularly and during sentinel events using an ACP and family meeting format. Lastly, integrating geriatric renal palliative care concepts is beneficial in caring for elderly patients with CKD by providing symptom management and helping with the difficult decisions and transitions of care that will arise during the clinical course of elderly patients with renal disease.

REFERENCES

1. Johansen KL, Chertow GM, Jin C, et al. Significance of frailty among dialysis patients. J Am Soc Nephrol 2007;18:2960–7.
2. Shlipak MG, Stehman-Breen C, Fried LF, et al. The presence of frailty in elderly persons with chronic renal insufficiency. Am J Kidney Dis 2004;43:861–7.
3. Fried LF, Lee JS, Shlipak M, et al. Chronic kidney disease and functional limitation in older people: health, aging and body composition study. J Am Geriatr Soc 2006;54:750–6.
4. Kurella M, Covinsky KE, Collins AJ, et al. Octogenarians and nonagenarians starting dialysis in the United States. Ann Intern Med 2007;146:177–83.
5. Couchoud C, Labeeuw M, Moranne O, et al. A clinical score to predict 6-month prognosis in elderly patients starting dialysis for end-stage renal disease. Nephrol Dial Transplant 2009;24:1553–61.
6. Murtagh FE, Marsh JE, Donohoe P, et al. Dialysis or not? A comparative survival study of patients over 75 years with chronic kidney disease stage 5. Nephrol Dial Transplant 2007;22:1955–62.
7. Cohen LM, Ruthazer R, Moss AH, et al. Predicting six-month mortality for patients who are on maintenance hemodialysis. Clin J Am Soc Nephrol 2010;5:72–9.
8. Jassal SV, Chiu E, Hladunewich M. Loss of independence in patients starting dialysis at 80 years of age or older. N Engl J Med 2009;361:1612–3.
9. Kurella M, Covinsky KE, Chertow GM, et al. Functional status of elderly adults before and after initiation of dialysis. N Engl J Med 2009;361:1539–47.
10. Lamping DL, Constantinovici N, Roderick P, et al. Clinical outcomes, quality of life, and costs in the North Thames Dialysis Study of elderly people on dialysis: a prospective cohort study. Lancet 2000;356:1543–50.
11. USRDS 2012 Annual Data Report: atlas of end-stage renal disease in the United States. National Institutes of Health, National Institute of Diabetes and Digestive and Kidney Diseases. Available at: http://www.usrds.org/atlas.aspx. Accessed February 12, 2013.
12. Kurella M, Chertow GM, Fried LF, et al. Chronic kidney disease and cognitive impairment in the elderly: the health, aging, and body composition study. J Am Soc Nephrol 2005;16:2127–33.
13. Griva K, Stygall J, Hankins M, et al. Cognitive impairment and 7-year mortality in dialysis patients. Am J Kidney Dis 2010;56:693–703.
14. Bao Y, Dalrymple L, Chertow GM, et al. Frailty, dialysis initiation, and mortality in end-stage renal disease. Arch Intern Med 2012;172:1071–7.
15. Fried LP, Tangen CM, Walston J, et al. Frailty in older adults: evidence for a phenotype. J Gerontol A Biol Sci Med Sci 2001;56:M146–56.

16. Swidler M. Chapter 37, Dialysis decisions in the elderly patient with advanced CKD and the role of nondialytictherapy. In: Oreopoulos D, Wiggins J, editors. American Society of Nephrology Geriatric Nephrology Curriculum. Washington, DC: American Society of Nephrology; 2009. http://www.asn-online.org/education/distancelearning/curricula/geriatrics/Chapter37.pdf. Accessed February 3, 2013.

17. Davison SN. End-of-life care preferences and needs: perceptions of patients with chronic kidney disease. Clin J Am Soc Nephrol 2010;5:195–204.

18. Moss AH. Ethical principles and processes guiding dialysis decision-making. Clin J Am Soc Nephrol 2011;6:2313–7.

19. Jonsen A, Siegler M, Winslade W. Clinical ethics: a practical approach to ethical decisions in medicine. 6th edition. New York: McGraw Hill; 2006.

20. Balducci L, Extermann M, Carreca I. Management of breast cancer in the older woman. Cancer Control 2001;8:431–41.

21. Hamerman D. Toward an understanding of frailty. Ann Intern Med 1999;130: 945–50.

22. Basso U, Monfardini S. Multidimensional geriatric evaluation in elderly cancer patients: a practical approach. Eur J Cancer Care 2004;13:424–33.

23. Rodin MB, Mohile SG. A practical approach to geriatric assessment in oncology. J Clin Oncol 2007;25:1936–44.

24. Swidler MA. Geriatric renal palliative care. J Gerontol 2012;67:1400–9.

25. Moss AH, Holley JL, Davison SN, et al. Core curriculum in nephrology. Palliative care. Am J Kidney Dis 2004;43:172–85.

26. Wong CF, McCarthy M, Williams PS. Factors affecting survival in advanced chronic kidney disease patients who choose not to receive dialysis. Ren Fail 2007;29:653–9.

27. Carson RC, Juszczack M, Davenport A, et al. Is maximum conservative management an equivalent treatment option to dialysis for elderly patients with significant comorbid disease? Clin J Am Soc Nephrol 2009;4:1611–9.

28. Holley JL. Palliative care in end-stage renal disease: focus on advance care planning, hospice referral, and bereavement. Semin Dial 2005;18:154–6.

29. Brown EA, Chambers EJ, Eggeling C. Palliative care in nephrology. Nephrol Dial Transplant 2008;23:789–91.

30. Moss AH. Revised dialysis clinical practice guideline promotes more informed decision-making. Clin J Am Soc Nephrol 2010;5:2380–3.

31. Lunney JR, Lynn J, Hogan C. Profiles of older Medicare decedents. J Am Geriatr Soc 2002;50:1108–12.

32. Lunney JR, Lynn J, Foley DJ, et al. Patterns of functional decline at the end of life. JAMA 2003;289:2387–92.

33. Murray SA, Kendall M, Boyd K, et al. Illness trajectories and palliative care. BMJ 2005;330:1007–11.

34. Murtagh F, Preston M, Higginson I. Patterns of dying: palliative care for non-malignant disease. Clin Med 2004;4:39–44.

35. Murtagh FE, Addington-Hall JM, Higginson IJ. End-stage renal disease: a new trajectory of functional decline in the last year of life. J Am Geriatr Soc 2011;59: 304–8.

36. Beddhu S, Bruns FJ, Saul M, et al. A simple comorbidity scale predicts clinical outcomes and costs in dialysis patients. Am J Med 2000;108:609–13.

37. Li M, Tomlinson G, Naglie G, et al. Geriatric comorbidities, such as falls, confer an independent mortality risk to elderly dialysis patients. Nephrol Dial Transplant 2008;23:1396–400.

38. Roshanravan B, Khatri M, Robinson-Cohen C, et al. A prospective study of frailty in nephrology-referred patients with CKD. Am J Kidney Dis 2012;60:912–21.

39. Letourneau I, Ouimet D, Dumont M, et al. Renal replacement in end-stage renal disease patients over 75 years old. Am J Nephrol 2003;23:71–7.

40. Moss AH, Ganjoo J, Sharma S, et al. Utility of the "surprise" question to identify dialysis patients with high mortality. Clin J Am Soc Nephrol 2008;3:1379–84.

41. Arias E. United States life tables, 2002. Natl Vital Stat Rep 2004;53:1–38.

42. Smith C, Da Silva-Gane M, Chandna S, et al. Choosing not to dialyse: evaluation of planned non-dialytic management in a cohort of patients with end-stage renal failure. Nephron Clin Pract 2003;95:c40–6.

43. Johnston S, Noble H. Factors influencing patients with stage 5 chronic kidney disease to opt for conservative management: a practitioner research study. J Clin Nurs 2011;21:1215–22.

44. Morton RL, Snelling P, Webster AC, et al. Factors influencing patient choice of dialysis versus conservative care to treat end-stage kidney disease. Can Med Assoc J 2012;185:E277–83.

45. Chandna SM, Da Silva-Gane M, Marshall C, et al. Survival of elderly patient with stage 5 CKD: comparison of conservative management and renal replacement therapy. Nephrol Dial Transplant 2011;26:1608–14.

46. Swidler MA. Palliative care and geriatric treatment of patients with advanced chronic kidney disease. In: Nephrology Self-Assessment Program (Neph-SAP):Geriatric Nephrology. Washington, DC. Clin J Am Soc Nephrol 2011; 10:67–80.

47. Holley J, Davison SN, Moss AH. Nephrologists' changing practices in reported end-of-life decision-making. Clin J Am Soc Nephrol 2007;2(1):107–11.

48. Davison SN. Pain in hemodialysis patients: prevalence, cause, severity and management. Am J Kidney Dis 2003;42:1239–47.

49. Weisbord SD, Fried LF, Mor MK, et al. Renal provider recognition of symptoms in patients on maintenance hemodialysis. Clin J Am Soc Nephrol 2007;2:960–7.

50. Weisbord SD, Fried LF, Arnold RM, et al. Prevalence, severity and importance of physical and emotional symptoms in chronic hemodialysis patients. J Am Soc Nephrol 2005;16:2487–94.

51. Weisbord SD, Carmody SS, Bruns FJ, et al. Symptom burden, quality of life, advance care planning and the potential value of palliative care in severely ill haemodialysis patients. Nephrol Dial Transplant 2003;18:1345–52.

52. O'Connor NR, Kumar P. Conservative management of end-stage renal disease without dialysis: a systemic review. J Palliat Med 2012;15:228–35.

53. Swartz RD, Perry E. Advance directives are associated with "good deaths" in chronic dialysis patients. J Am Soc Nephrol 1993;3:1623–30.

54. Murray AH, Arko C, Chen SC, et al. Use of hospice in the United States dialysis population. Clin J Am Soc Nephrol 2006;1:1248–55.

55. Wong SP, Kreuter W, O'Hare AM. Treatment intensity at the end of life in older adults receiving long-term dialysis. Arch Intern Med 2012;172:661–2.

56. Chater S, Davison S, Germain M, et al. Withdrawal from dialysis: a palliative care perspective. Clin Nephrol 2006;66:364–72.

Drug Dosing in Elderly Patients with Chronic Kidney Disease

Jessica Lassiter, PharmD, BCPS[a], William M. Bennett, MD[b],
Ali J. Olyaei, PharmD[c],*

KEYWORDS

- Elderly • Medication • Chronic kidney disease • Health care cost

KEY POINTS

- An optimal balance between improved outcomes while minimizing potential for drug toxicity is essential in patients with Chronic Kidney Disease.
- Correct assessment of kidney function is essential for determining drug dosing in the elderly with impaired renal function.
- For most drugs maintenance doses often require adjustment in elderly patients and those with CKD.

INTRODUCTION

The human body shows progressive decline in health and function and these changes are predictive of increased morbidity and mortality in the geriatric population.[1] As life expectancy continues to increase, the geriatric population will demand a large portion of health care resources including the use of prescription medications (**Fig. 1**). It is estimated that 80% of the geriatric population report regularly using prescription medications, nearly double the reported usage in those less than 65 years of age. Between 1992 and 2008, the average prescription drug costs for Medicare enrollees more than 65 years of age increased from approximately $600 to more than $2800 per year.[2] The growing health care costs among geriatric patients puts greater pressure on providers for judicious prescribing in this population.

Safe medication prescribing in the elderly, although important, can be difficult due to a multitude of factors such as comorbid conditions, larger quantity of medications, altered pharmacokinetics, and increased risk of mortality. Many of the landmark drug

[a] Department of Pharmacy Services, University of Michigan Hospital and Health Systems, Ann Arbor, MI, USA; [b] Clinical Transplant, Northwest Renal Clinic, Legacy Good Samaritan Hospital Transplant Services, Portland, OR, USA; [c] Division of Nephrology & Hypertension, Oregon State University and Oregon Health & Sciences University, 3303 Southwest Bond Avenue, CH12C, Portland, OR 97239, USA
* Corresponding author.
E-mail address: olyaeia@ohsu.edu

Clin Geriatr Med 29 (2013) 657–705
http://dx.doi.org/10.1016/j.cger.2013.05.008
0749-0690/13/$ – see front matter © 2013 Elsevier Inc. All rights reserved.

geriatric.theclinics.com

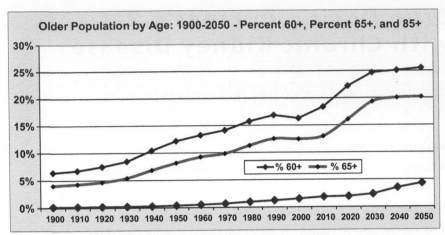

Fig. 1. Older population by age: 1900–2050. Percent 60+ years, 65+ years, and 85+ years. (*Data from* Projections of the population by age and sex for the United States: 2010 to 2050 (NP2008-T12). Population Division, US Census Bureau. Release date: August 14, 2008; Table 12.)

efficacy trials exclude patients greater than 65 years of age. From 2010 census data, nearly 25% of people in the United States more than 65 years of age report fair to poor health. Of Medicare beneficiaries greater than 65 years of age, nearly half have more than 3 chronic diseases and of these, 21% have more than 5 chronic diseases. Not surprisingly, chronic disease is a strong predictor for increased medication use and nursing home patients have been reported to be on from 3 to more than 10 medications per day.[3] In addition, approximately 65% to 70% of men and 70% to 80% of women in this age group are reported to have hypertension and 25% with diabetes. These 2 conditions account for almost half of the diagnoses leading to chronic kidney disease (CKD).

However, because of lack of evidence in the older population, proven therapies among younger populations may be underused. In addition, the high risk of drug interactions and adverse events make many therapies contraindicated in geriatric patients.

A delicate balance must be made regarding risk reduction for sequelae of disease and the increased potential for adverse events in the elderly. In addition to a larger number of medications, especially in patients with CKD, pharmacokinetic and pharmacodynamics changes that occur with age must be taken into consideration. For example, studies targeting blood pressure reduction in the elderly have shown reduction in systolic blood pressure leads to a decrease risk for stroke and major cardiac events. However, the target systolic blood pressure ranges may be adjusted for these patients because the risk of orthostasis and falls must be considered.[4,5] Adverse events in elderly patients on multiple medications may be mistaken for new onset or progression of disease.[6,7] The addition of anticholinergic medications, for example, frequently causes altered mental status in the elderly. Changes in mental status could be mistaken as progression of decline in cognitive status or progression of dementia. These events are often 3-fold to 10-fold higher in the elderly with CKD.[8]

A study done by Lindeman and colleagues[9] demonstrated an age-related decrease in glomerular filtration rate (GFR). Because many medications or their metabolites are filtered through the kidney, patients with CKD are prone to increased exposure to active drug.[7] In addition, hepatic changes associated with age may increase serum drug levels and prolong the half-life of medications undergoing hepatic metabolism.[10–12] For instance, medications such as morphine are primarily metabolized in the liver but have renally excreted active metabolites.[13] The combination of age-related changes and the presence of CKD may increase the risk for accumulation of drug and the potential for adverse outcomes.[14,15] Careful medication selection using patient-specific markers is necessary for safe prescribing in the elderly.

A useful method of assessing drug dosing in the elderly is to estimate the GFR.[16] Appropriate dose adjustment of medications can prevent potential toxicity to the kidneys or other adverse effects. Age-related changes to the kidneys increase their susceptibility to toxicity and reduce the ability for recovery after injury. The most accurate assessment of GFR is measured through 24-hour urine collection with infusion of an exogenous substance such as inulin.[17] Because of the cost and difficulty obtaining these data for the average patient, regression equations have been developed using serum creatinine (SCr) level as a marker for clearance. Initially creatinine clearance was calculated using the Cockcroft-Gault (CG) method. However, this equation was developed using a homogenous population and was not validated in the elderly. In recent years, 2 equations have been developed using larger populations for more accurate assessment of estimated GFR (eGFR), the Modification of Diet in Renal Disease (MDRD) equation and the CKD Epidemiology Collaboration (CKD-EPI) equation.[16,18–20] Despite improvements in accurate assessment of renal function, SCr level is an imperfect marker of kidney function, particularly in the elderly. Concomitant medications may falsely increase SCr by interfering with secretion, whereas others may increase metabolic load by increasing creatinine production. Low muscle mass or malnutrition, common among the elderly population, may also affect SCr and thus assessment of eGFR.[21]

APPROACH TO DOSAGE ADJUSTMENT IN OLDER ADULTS

The focus should be placed on reaching the optimal balance between improved outcomes while minimizing potential for drug toxicity. The adage start low and go slow is essential in the elderly. The following recommendations offer guidance for achieving safe prescribing in the elderly patient with CKD. Patient-specific factors such as comorbid conditions and drug interactions should always be considered.

Step 1: Medical History and Physical Examination

A complete medical history and physical examination provides baseline information for medication prescribing. In patients with kidney disease, determining the cause and duration of dysfunction is important. It can offer insight into whether they are currently stable or in an acute or acute on chronic process. Volume status should also be assessed, particularly in patients with kidney disease. Shifts in intracellular and extracellular fluid balance can alter the volume of distribution of many drugs. A sedentary lifestyle can lead to decreased muscle mass and increased fat stores in older adults, leading to change in the distribution of hydrophilic agents. In addition, age-related decreases in total body water and thus a reduction in blood volume should also be considered.[22] Medications with a small volume of distribution and narrow therapeutic window such as aminoglycosides are examples of agents greatly affected by seemingly small shifts in extracellular volume. Combined with this, hepatic changes may further alter drug kinetics in the elderly. Decreasing efficiency in phase I hepatic metabolism may alter drug levels and the half-life of medications.[3] Medications such as verapamil and diltiazem can reduce metabolism in the older population, causing increased effect.

Drug allergies and intolerances can assist in the selection of future treatment modalities. Coexisting conditions are important to evaluate the usefulness and efficacy of drug regimens. A review of medications for potential interactions or nephrotoxic exposure is important because older adults often see several providers and medication lists may be inaccurate and incomplete.[23]

Step 2: Assessment of Kidney Function

Assessment of kidney function is essential for determining drug dosing in the elderly. Many medications are renally cleared, therefore accurate estimation of GFR is important for selecting appropriate dosing when initiating a new medication. Several equations have been studied and validated as estimations of GFR. Previously, the CG formula was the primary method for estimating GFR by calculating creatinine clearance.[17] In addition, pharmacokinetic studies of new medications were based on renal function assessments using the CG formula. The equation includes variables of age in years, ideal body weight (IBW; kg), and SCr (mg/dL).

IBW may be calculated from

IBW (men): 50.0 kg + 2.3 kg for every 2.5 cm over 152 cm
IBW (women): 45.5 kg + 2.3 kg for every 2.5 cm over 152 cm

The CG formula is

$$CrCl = \frac{(140 - age) \times IBW}{72 \times SCr}$$

where CrCl is creatinine clearance. Multiply the result by 0.85 for women.

Although still widely used, further studies have shown that the CG formula is inaccurate in certain populations, including the elderly.[24] More recently, 2 equations have been developed for estimating GFR and have been validated in large population-based studies. The first is the 4-variable MDRD equation. This equation has now been widely accepted as the standard for assessment of eGFR. The US Food and Drug Administration has recommended the use of MDRD in conjunction with CG for any pharmacokinetic studies being conducted.[25] Using variables for age, sex, SCr, and race, the MDRD equation calculates eGFR[26]:

$$eGFR = 175 \times SCr^{-1.154} \times age^{-0.203} \times 1.212 \text{ (if black)} \times 0.742 \text{ (if female)}$$

The second equation for calculating eGFR is the CKD-EPI equation. Using similar variables as MDRD, the equation also calculates eGFR:

$$eGFR = 141 \times \min\left(\frac{SCr}{k, 1}\right)^{\alpha} \times \max\left(\frac{SCr}{k, 1}\right)^{-1.209} \times 0.993^{age} \times 1.018 \text{ (if female)}$$
$$\times 1.159 \text{ (if black)}$$

where k is 0.7 for women and 0.9 for men, α is −0.329 for women and −0.411 for men, min indicates the minimum of SCr/k or 1, and max indicates the maximum of SCr/k or 1.

In comparisons between the CG, MDRD, and CKD-EPI in the elderly, MDRD and CKD-EPI have been shown to more accurately assess eGFR than CG. In a further study between the MDRD and CKD-EPI equations, at higher eGFR (eGFR >60 mL/min) CKD-EPI outperforms MDRD.[27] However, in the elderly with lower GFR, MDRD and CKD-EPI are not statistically different. Studies are being conducted to develop more precise equations for the assessment of renal function in the elderly. One such study, conducted in Germany, used cystatin C as a marker for renal function. The equation shows promise for decreasing the potential for overestimation or underestimation of GFR, however further studies are necessary to assess its widespread use.

Despite the usefulness of these equations, patient characteristics must also be assessed. Each equation uses SCr as the primary biomarker of eGFR. Although useful, SCr is subject to variance due to factors such as decreases in muscle mass, changes in protein intake (or malnutrition), and false increase caused by medications blocking secretion (ie, cimetidine or trimethoprim).[11,28] SCr as a marker in acute kidney injury is also inaccurate. The lag time between injury onset and increase in SCr creates significant discordance between actual function and calculated eGFR using SCr. Consideration of timing and urine output is important for appropriate drug dosing in these situations.

Step 3: Loading Dose Determination

Loading doses of medications are often used as a method of reaching the steady state of a drug more rapidly when early treatment is essential. Antibiotics are an example where timeliness is essential for proper treatment of infection. Steady state is reached after approximately 5 half-lives. The half-life of medications is often prolonged in the elderly, particularly in those with CKD. Loading doses can assist in shortening the time to steady state in these populations. They may be calculated using the following equation:

$$LD = Vd \times IBW \times [Cp]$$

where Vd is the volume of distribution in L/kg, IBW in kg, and Cp is the desired plasma concentration in mg/L.

As a general rule, loading doses of medications should not be adjusted based on kidney or liver disease. However, a few agents do require smaller loading doses because of altered volume of distribution in patients with CKD. The primary example is digoxin. Loading doses of digoxin are decreased by 50% in patients with end-stage renal disease (ESRD) to reduce the risk for toxicity as the drug accumulates over time.

Step 4: Maintenance Dose Determination

Unlike loading doses, maintenance doses often require adjustment in elderly patients and those with CKD. Medications that are excreted unchanged or have active metabolites that are excreted through the kidney require dose changes for prevention of toxicity. Modifications in dosing for the elderly may be accomplished by reduction in dose, by extending the interval, or both. For example, morphine, although metabolized through the liver, is excreted along with its active metabolites through the kidney. Regular dosing of this medication in severe kidney disease allows for accumulation of active drug and potential adverse effects. However, when used intermittently, morphine is safe in patients with lower GFR. For medications requiring adequate peak or trough concentrations such as aminoglycosides, altering the interval is generally successful in reaching efficacy while preventing toxicity by allowing adequate clearance of the drug. For most drugs, a combination of interval extension and dose reduction is necessary.

Table 1
Equations based on serum creatinine assays in adults that are not traceable to the standard reference material

Study, Year, Reference	Equation Name	Expression	Formula
Cockcroft & Gault,[17] 1976	CG	CrCl in mL/min	$CrCl = \dfrac{(140 - age) \times weight}{72 \times SCr}$ (×0.85 if female) SCr in mg/dL
Levey et al,[29] 2006	4-variable MDRD	GFR in mL/min per 1.73 m²	$eGFR = 186 \times SCr^{-1.154} \times age^{-0.203} \times 0.742$ (if female) SCr in mg/dL
Levey et al,[30] 1999	6-variable MDRD	GFR in mL/min per 1.73 m²	$eGFR = 170 \times SCr^{-0.999} \times age^{-0.176} \times 1.180$ (if black) $\times 0.762$ (if female) $\times BUN^{-0.170} \times albumin^{0.318}$ SCr in mg/dL, blood urea nitrogen in mg/dL, and albumin in g/dL
Levey et al,[18] 2009	CKD-EPI	GFR in mL/min per 1.73 m²	$eGFR = 141 \times \min\left(\dfrac{SCr}{k}, 1\right)^{\alpha} \times \max\left(\dfrac{SCr}{k}, 1\right)^{-1.209} \times 0.993^{age} \times 1.018$ (if female) $\times 1.159$ (if black) SCr in mg/dL

Table 2
Therapeutics Drug Monitoring in CKD patients

	Therapeutic Range	When to Draw Sample	How Often to Draw Levels
Aminoglycosides (conventional dosing): gentamicin, tobramycin, amikacin	Gentamicin and tobramycin: Trough: 0.5–2 mg/L Peak: 5–8 mg/L Amikacin: Peak: 20–30 mg/L Trough: <10 mg/L	Obtain drug level 30 min before and after dose Peak: 30 min after a 30–45 min infusion	Check peak and trough with third dose For therapy less than 72 h, levels not necessary. Repeat drug levels weekly or if renal function changes
Aminoglycosides (24-h dosing): gentamicin, tobramycin, amikacin	0.5–3 mg/L	Obtain random drug level 12 h after dose	After initial dose. Repeat drug level in 1 wk or if renal function changes
Carbamazepine	4–12 µg/mL	Trough: immediately before dosing	Check 2–4 d after first dose or change in dose
Cyclosporin	150–400 ng/mL	Trough: immediately before dosing	Daily for first week, then weekly
Digoxin	0.8–2.0 ng/mL	23 h after maintenance dose	5–7 d after first dose for patients with normal renal and hepatic function; 15–20 d in anephric patients
Lidocaine	1–5 µg/mL	8 h after intravenous infusion started or changed	
Lithium	Acute: 0.8–1.2 mmol/L Chronic: 0.6–0.8 mmol/L	Trough: Before AM dose, at least 12 h since last dose	

(continued on next page)

Table 2
(continued)

	Therapeutic Range	When to Draw Sample	How Often to Draw Levels
Phenobarbital	15–40 µg/mL	Trough: immediately before dosing	Check 2 wk after first dose or change in dose. Follow-up level in 1–2 mo
Phenytoin	10–20 µg/mL	Trough: immediately before dosing	5–7 d after first dose or after change in dose
Free phenytoin	1–2 µg/mL		
Procainamide	4–10 µg/mL	Trough: immediately before next dose or 12–18 h after starting or changing an infusion	
n-Acetyl procainamide, a procainamide metabolite	Trough: 4 µg/mL Peak: 8 µg/mL 10–30 µg/mL	Draw with procainamide sample	
Quinidine	1–5 µg/mL	Trough: immediately before next dose	
Sirolimus	10–20 ng/dL	Trough: immediately before next dose	
Tacrolimus (FK-506)	10–15 ng/mL	Trough: immediately before next dose	Daily for first week, then weekly
Theophylline by mouth or aminophylline intravenously	15–20 µg/mL	Trough: immediately before next dose	
Valproic acid (divalproex sodium)	40–100 µg/mL	Trough: immediately before next dose	Check 2–4 d after first dose or change in dose
Vancomycin	Trough: 5–15 mg/L Peak: 25–40 mg/L	Trough: immediately before dose Peak: 60 min after a 60-min infusion	With third dose (when initially starting therapy, or after each dosage adjustment). For therapy less than 72 h, levels not necessary. Repeat drug levels if renal function changes

Table 3
Antimicrobial dosing in renal failure

Drugs	Normal Dosage	% of Renal Excretion	Dosage Adjustment in Renal Failure			Comments
			GFR >50 mL/min	GFR 10–50 mL/min	GFR <10 mL/min	
Aminoglycoside antibiotics						Nephrotoxic. Ototoxic. Toxicity worse when hyperbilirubinemic. Measure serum levels for efficacy and toxicity. Peritoneal absorption increases with presence of inflammation. Vd increases with edema, obesity, and ascites
Streptomycin	7.5 mg/kg every 12 h (1.0 g every 24 h for tuberculosis)	60%	Every 24 h	Every 24–72 h	Every 72–96 h	For the treatment of tuberculosis. May be less nephrotoxic than other members of class
Kanamycin	7.5 mg/kg every 8 h	50%–90%	60%–90% every 12 h or 100% every 12–24 h	30%–70% every 12–18 h or 100% every 24–48 h	20%–30% every 24–48 h or 100% every 48–72 h	Nephrotoxic. Ototoxic. Toxicity worse when hyperbilirubinemic. Vd increases with edema, obesity, and ascites. Do not use once-daily dosing in patients with CrCl less than 30–40 mL/min or in patients with acute renal failure or uncertain level of kidney function
Gentamicin	1.7 mg/kg every 8 h	95%	60%–90% every 8–12 h or 100% every 12–24 h	30%–70% every 12 h or 100% every 24–48 h	20%–30% every 24–48 h or 100% every 48–72 h	Concurrent penicillins may result in subtherapeutic aminoglycoside levels Peak: 6–8 mcg/ml Trough: <2 mcg/ml

(continued on next page)

Table 3
(continued)

| Drugs | Normal Dosage | % of Renal Excretion | Dosage Adjustment in Renal Failure | | | Comments |
			GFR >50 mL/min	GFR 10–50 mL/min	GFR <10 mL/min	
Tobramicin	1.7 mg/kg every 8 h	95%	60%–90% every 8–12 h or 100% every 12–24 h	30%–70% every 12 h or 100% every 24–48 h	20%–30% every 24–48 h or 100% every 48–72 h	Concurrent penicillins may result in subtherapeutic aminoglycoside levels Peak: 6–8 Trough: <2
Netilmicin	2 mg/kg every 8 h	95%	50%–90% every 8–12 h or 100% every 12–24 h	20%–60% every 12 h or 100% every 24–48 h	10%–20% every 24–48 h or 100% every 48–72	May be less ototoxic than other members of class Peak: 6–8 Trough: <2
Amikacin	7.5 mg/kg every 12 h	95%	60%–90% every 12 h or 100% every 12–24 h	30%–70% every 12–18 h or 100% every 24–48 h	20%–30% every 24–48 h or 100% every 48–72 h	Monitor levels Peak: 20–30 Trough: <5
Cephalosporin						Coagulation abnormalities Transitory increase in blood urea nitrogen, rash, and serum sickness-like syndrome
Oral Cephalosporins						
Cefaclor	250–500 mg 3 times a day	70%	100%	100%	50%	
Cefadroxil	500 to 1 g 2 times a day	80%	100%	100%	50%	
Cefixime	200–400 mg every 12 h	85%	100%	100%	50%	
Cefpodoxime	200 mg every 12 h	30%	100%	100%	100%	
Ceftibuten	400 mg every 24 h	70%	100%	100%	50%	
Cefuroxime axetil	250–500 mg 3 times a day	90%	100%	100%	100%	Malabsorbed in presence of H2 blockers. Absorbed better with food

					Comments
Cephalexin	250–500 mg 3 times a day	95%	100%	100%	100%	Rare allergic interstitial nephritis. Absorbed well when given intraperitoneally. May cause bleeding from impaired prothrombin biosynthesis
Cephradine	250–500 mg 3 times a day	100%	100%	100%	50%	Rare allergic interstitial nephritis. Absorbed well when given intraperitoneally. May cause bleeding from impaired prothrombin biosynthesis

Intravenous Cephalosporins

						Comments
Cefamandole	1–2 g intravenously every 6–8 h	100%	Every 6 h	Every 8 h	Every 12 h	
Cefazolin	1–2 g intravenously every 8 h	80%	Every 8 h	Every 12 h	Every 12–24 h	
Cefepime	1–2 g intravenously every 8 h	85%	Every 8–12 h	Every 12 h	Every 24 h	
Cefmetazole	1–2 g intravenously every 8 h	85%	Every 8 h	Every 12 h	Every 24 h	
Cefoperazone	1–2 g intravenously every 12 h	20%	No renal adjustment is required			Displaced from protein by bilirubin. Reduce dose by 50% for jaundice. May prolong prothrombin time
Cefotaxime	1–2 g intravenously every 6–8 h	60%	Every 8 h	Every 12 h	Every 12–24 h	Active metabolite in ESRD. Reduce dose further for combined hepatic and renal failure
Cefotetan	1–2 g intravenously every 12 h	75%	Every 12 h	Every 12–24 h	Every 24 h	

(continued on next page)

Table 3
(continued)

Drugs	Normal Dosage	% of Renal Excretion	Dosage Adjustment in Renal Failure			Comments
			GFR >50 mL/min	GFR 10–50 mL/min	GFR <10 mL/min	
Cefoxitin	1–2 g intravenously every 6 h	80%	Every 6 h	Every 8–12 h	Every 12 h	May produce false increase in SCr by interference with assay
Ceftazidime	1–2 g intravenously every 8 h	70%	Every 8 h	Every 12 h	Every 24 h	
Ceftriaxone	1–2 g intravenously every 24 h	50%	No renal adjustment is required			
Cefuroxime sodium	0.75–1.5 g intravenously every 8 h	90%	Every 8 h	Every 8–12 h	Every 12–24 h	Rare allergic interstitial nephritis. Absorbed well when given intraperitoneally. May cause bleeding from impaired prothrombin biosynthesis
Penicillin						Bleeding abnormalities, hypersensitivity, seizures
Oral Penicillins						
Amoxicillin	500 mg by mouth 3 times a day	60%	100%	100%	50%–75%	
Ampicillin	500 mg by mouth every 6 h	60%	100%	100%	50%–75%	
Dicloxacillin	250–500 mg by mouth every 6 h	50%	100%	100%	50%–75%	
Penicillin V	250–500 mg by mouth every 6 h	70%	100%	100%	50%–75%	
Intravenous Penicillins						
Ampicillin	1–2 g intravenously every 6 h	60%	Every 6 h	Every 8 h	Every 12 h	

Drug	Dose					Comments
Nafcillin	1–2 g intravenously every 4 h	35%	No renal adjustment is required			
Penicillin G	2–3 million units intravenously every 4 h	70%	Every 4–6 h	Every 6 h	Every 8 h	Seizures. False-positive urine protein reactions. Six million units/d upper limit dose in ESRD
Piperacillin	3–4 g intravenously every 4–6 h		No renal adjustment is required			Specific toxicity: sodium, 1.9 mEq/g
Ticarcillin/ clavulanate	3.1 g intravenously every 4–6 h	85%	1–2 g every 4 h	1–2 g every 8 h	1–2 g every 12 h	Specific toxicity: sodium, 5.2 mEq/g
Piperacillin/ tazobactam	3.375 g intravenously every 6–8 h	75%–90%	Every 4–6 h	Every 6–8 h	Every 8 h	Specific toxicity: sodium, 1.9 mEq/g
Quinolones						Photosensitivity, food, dairy products, tube feeding and Al(OH)$_3$ may decrease the absorption of quinolones
Cinoxacin	500 mg every 12 h	55%	100%	50%	Avoid	
Fleroxacin	400 mg every 12 h	70%	100%	50%–75%	50%	
Ciprofloxacin	200–400 mg intravenously every 24 h	60%	Every 12 h	Every 12–24 h	Every 24 h	Poorly absorbed with antacids, sucralfate, and phosphate binders. Intravenous dose one-third of oral dose. Decreases phenytoin levels
Lomefloxacin	400 mg every 24 h	76%	100%	200–400 mg every 48 h	50%	Agents in this group are malabsorbed in the presence of magnesium, calcium, aluminum, and iron. Theophylline metabolism is impaired. Higher oral doses may be needed to treat peritonitis due to continuous ambulatory peritoneal dialysis

(continued on next page)

Table 3
(continued)

Drugs	Normal Dosage	% of Renal Excretion	Dosage Adjustment in Renal Failure			Comments
			GFR >50 mL/min	GFR 10–50 mL/min	GFR <10 mL/min	
Levofloxacin	500 mg by mouth every day	70%	Every 12 h	250 every 12 h	250 every 12 h	L-Isomer of ofloxacin: seems to have similar pharmacokinetics and toxicities
Moxifloxacin	400 mg every day	20%	No renal adjustment is required			
Nalidixic acid	1.0 g every 6 h	High	100%	Avoid	Avoid	Agents in this group are malabsorbed in the presence of magnesium, calcium, aluminum, and iron. Theophylline metabolism is impaired. Higher oral doses may be needed to treat peritonitis due to continuous ambulatory peritoneal dialysis
Norfloxacin	400 mg by mouth every 12 h	30%	Every 12 h	Every 12–24 h	Every 24 h	See above
Ofloxacin	200–400 mg by mouth every 12 h	70%	Every 12 h	Every 12–24 h	Every 24 h	See above
Pefloxacin	400 mg every 24 h	11%	100%	100%	100%	Excellent bidirectional transperitoneal movement
Sparfloxacin	400 mg every 24 h	10%	100%	50%–75%	50% every 48 h	
Trovafloxacin	200–300 mg by mouth every 12 h	10%	No renal adjustment is required			
Miscellaneous Agents						
Azithromycin	250–500 mg by mouth every day	6%	No renal adjustment is required			No drug-drug interaction with cyclosporine and tacrolimus (CSA/FK)

Drug	Dose	%	Adjustment 1	Adjustment 2	Adjustment 3	Comments
Clarithromycin	500 mg by mouth 2 times a day	20%				Increase CSA/FK level
Clindamycin	150–450 mg by mouth 3 times a day	10%	No renal adjustment is required			
Dirithromycin	500 mg by mouth every day		No renal adjustment is required			Nonenzymatically hydrolyzed to active compound erythomycylamine
Erythromycin	250–500 mg by mouth 4 times a day	15%	No renal adjustment is required			Increase CSA/FK level, avoid in transplant patients
Imipenem/ cilastatin	250–500 mg intravenously every 6 h	50%	500 mg every 8 h	250–500 every 8–12 h	250 mg every 12 h	Seizures in ESRD. Nonrenal clearance in acute renal failure is less than in chronic renal failure. Administered with cilastin to prevent nephrotoxicity of renal metabolite
Meropenem	1 g intravenously every 8 h	65%	1 g every 8 h	0.5–1 g every 12 h	0.5–1 g every 24 h	
Metronidazole	500 mg intravenously every 6 h	20%	No renal adjustment is required			Peripheral neuropathy, increased liver function tests, disulfiram reaction with alcoholic beverages
Pentamidine	4 mg/kg/d	5%	Every 24 h	Every 24 h	Every 48 h	Inhalation may cause bronchospasm, intravenous administration may cause hypotension, hypoglycemia, and nephrotoxicity
Trimethoprim/ sulfamethoxazole	800/160 mg by mouth 2 times a day	70%	Every 12 h	Every 18 h	Every 24 h	Increase serum creatinine. Can cause hyperkalemia

(continued on next page)

Table 3
(continued)

Drugs	Normal Dosage	% of Renal Excretion	Dosage Adjustment in Renal Failure			Comments
			GFR >50 mL/min	GFR 10–50 mL/min	GFR <10 mL/min	
Vancomycin	1 g intravenously every 12 h	90%	Every 12 h	Every 24–36 h	Every 48–72 h	Nephrotoxic, ototoxic, may prolong the neuromuscular blockade effect of muscle relaxants. Peak: 30, trough 5–10
Vancomycin	125–250 mg by mouth 4 times a day	0%	100%	100%	100%	Oral vancomycin is indicated only for the treatment of *Clostridium difficile*
Antituberculosis Antibiotics						
Rifampin	300–600 mg by mouth every day	20%	No renal adjustment is required			Decrease CSA/FK level. Many drug interactions
Antifungal Agents						
Amphotericin B	0.5 mg–1.5 mg/kg/d	<1%	No renal adjustment is required			Nephrotoxic, infusion related reactions, give 250 mL of normal saline before each dose
Amphotec	4–6 mg/kg/d	<1%	No renal adjustment is required			
Abelcet	5 mg/kg/d	<1%	No renal adjustment is required			
AmBisome	3–5 mg/kg/d	<1%	No renal adjustment is required			
Azoles and Other Antifungals						
Fluconazole	200–800 mg intravenously every day/2 times a day	70%	100%	100%	50%	Increase CSA/FK level
Flucytosine	37.5 mg/kg	90%	Every 12 h	Every 16 h	Every 24 h	Hepatic dysfunction. Marrow suppression more common in azotemic patients

Griseofulvin	125–250 mg every 6 h	1%	100%	100%	100%	
Itraconazole	200 mg every 12 h	35%	100%	100%	50%	Poor oral absorption
Ketoconazole	200–400 mg by mouth every day	15%	100%	100%	100%	Hepatotoxic
Miconazole	1200–3600 mg/d	1%	100%	100%	100%	
Terbinafine	250 mg by mouth every day	>1%	100%	100%	100%	
Voriconazole	4 mg/kg every 12 h	>1%	100%	100%	100%	Intravenous use should be limited to only a few doses in patients with CrCl <30 mL/min
Antiviral Agents						
Acyclovir	200–800 mg by mouth 5 times/d	50%	100%	100%	50%	Poor absorption. Neurotoxicity in ESRD. Intravenous preparation can cause renal failure if injected rapidly
Adefovir	10 mg	45%	100%	10 mg every 48 h	10 mg every 72 h	Nephrotoxic
Amantadine	100–200 mg every 12 h	90%	100%	50%	25%	
Cidofovir	5 mg/kg weekly ×2 (induction), 5 mg/kg every 2 wk	90%	No data. Avoid	No data. Avoid	No data. Avoid	Dose-limiting nephrotoxicity with proteinuria, glycosuria, renal insufficiency, nephrotoxicity, and renal clearance reduced with coadministration of probenecid
Delavirdine	400 mg every 8 h	5%	No data: 100%	No data: 100%	No data: 100%	
Didanosine	200 mg every 12 h (125 mg if <60 kg)	40%–69%	Every 12 h	Every 24 h	50% every 24 h	Pancreatitis

(continued on next page)

Table 3
(continued)

Drugs	Normal Dosage	% of Renal Excretion	Dosage Adjustment in Renal Failure			Comments
			GFR >50 mL/min	GFR 10–50 mL/min	GFR <10 mL/min	
Famciclovir	250–500 mg by mouth 2 times a day to 3 times a day	60%	Every 8 h	Every 12 h	Every 24 h	Varicella-zoster virus: 500 mg by mouth 3 times a day Herpes simplex virus: 250 by mouth 2 times a day. Metabolized to active compound penciclovir
Foscarnet	40–80 mg intravenously every 8 h	85%	40–20 mg every 8–24 h according to ClCr			Nephrotoxic, neurotoxic, hypocalcemia, hypophosphatemia, hypomagnesemia, and hypokalemia
Ganciclovir intravenously	5 mg/kg every 12 h	95%	Every 12 h	Every 24 h	2,5 mg/kg every day	Granulocytopenia and thrombocytopenia
Ganciclovir by mouth	1000 mg by mouth 3 times a day	95%	1000 mg 3 times a day	1000 mg 2 times a day	1000 mg every day	Oral ganciclovir should be used ONLY for prevention of cytomegalovirus infection. Always use intravenous ganciclovir for the treatment of cytomegalovirus infection
Indinavir	800 mg every 8 h	10%	No data: 100%	No data: 100%	No data: 100%	Nephrolithiasis, acute renal failure caused by crystalluria, tubulointerstitial nephritis
Lamivudine	150 mg by mouth 2 times a day	80%	Every 12 h	Every 24 h	50 mg every 24 h	For hepatitis B

Drug	Dose					Comments
Nelfinavir	750 mg every 8 h	No data	No data	No data	No data	
Nevirapine	200 mg every 24 h for 14 d	<3%	No data: 100%	No data: 100%	No data: 100%	May be partially cleared by hemodialysis and peritoneal dialysis
Ribavirin	500–600 mg every 12 h	30%	100%	100%	50%	Hemolytic uremic syndrome
Rifabutin	300 mg every 24 h	5%–10%	100%	100%	100%	
Rimantadine	100 mg by mouth 2 times a day	25%	100%	100%	50%	
Ritonavir	600 mg every 12 h	3.50%	No data: 100%	No data: 100%	No data: 100%	Many drug interactions
Saquinavir	600 mg every 8 h	<4%	No data: 100%	No data: 100%	No data: 100%	
Stavudine	30–40 mg every 12 h	35%–40%	100%	50% every 12–24 h	50% every 24 h	
Valacyclovir	500–1000 mg every 8 h	50%	100%	50%	25%	Thrombotic thrombocytopenic purpura/hemolytic uremic syndrome
Vidarabine	15 mg/kg infusion every 24 h	50%	100%	100%	75%	
Zanamivir	2 puffs 2 times a day for 5 d	1%	100%	100%	100%	Bioavailability from inhalation and systemic exposure to drug is low
Zalcitabine	0.75 mg every 8 h	75%	100%	Every 12 h	Every 24 h	
Zidovudine	200 mg every 8 h, 300 mg every 12 h	8%–25%	100%	100%	100 mg every 8 h	Enormous interpatient variation. Metabolite renally excreted

Table 4
Analgesic drug dosing in renal failure

Analgesics	Normal Dosage	% of Renal Excretion	Dosage Adjustment in Renal Failure			Comments
			GFR >50 mL/min	GFR 10–50 mL/min	GFR <10 mL/min	
Narcotics and Narcotic Antagonists						
Alfentanil	Anesthetic induction 8–40 µg/kg	Hepatic	100%	100%	100%	Titrate the dose regimen
Butorphanol	2 mg every 3–4 h	Hepatic	100%	75%	50%	
Codeine	30–60 mg every 4–6 h	Hepatic	100%	75%	50%	
Fentanyl	Anesthetic induction (individualized)	Hepatic	100%	75%	50%	Continuous renal replacement therapy, titrate
Meperidine	50–100 mg every 3–4 h	Hepatic	100%	Avoid	Avoid	Normeperidine, an active metabolite, accumulates in ESRD and may cause seizures. Protein binding is reduced in ESRD. 20%–25% excreted unchanged in acidic urine
Methadone	2.5–5 mg every 6–8 h	Hepatic	100%	100%	50%–75%	Should not be used for acute pain
Morphine	20–25 mg every 4 h	Hepatic	100%	75%	50%	Increased sensitivity to drug effect in ESRD. Active metabolites
Naloxone	2 mg intravenously	Hepatic	100%	100%	100%	
Pentazocine	50 mg every 4 h	Hepatic	100%	75%	75%	
Propoxyphene	65 mg by mouth every 6–8 h	Hepatic	100%	100%	Avoid	Active metabolite norpropoxyphene accumulates in ESRD Cardiotoxic
Sufentanil	Anesthetic induction	Hepatic	100%	100%	100%	Continuous renal replacement therapy, titrate
Nonnarcotics						
Acetaminophen	650 mg every 4 h	Hepatic	Every 4 h	Every 6 h	Every 8 h	Overdose may be nephrotoxic. Drug is major metabolite of phenacetin
Acetylsalicylic acid	650 mg every 4 h	Hepatic (renal)	Every 4 h	Every 4–6 h	Avoid	Nephrotoxic in high doses. May decrease GFR when renal blood flow is prostaglandin dependent. May add to uremic gastrointestinal and hematologic symptoms. Protein binding reduced in ESRD

Table 5
Antihypertensive and cardiovascular agent dosing in renal failure

Antihypertensive and Cardiovascular Agents	Normal Dosage	% of Renal Excretion	Dosage Adjustment in Renal Failure			Comments
			GFR >50 mL/min	GFR 10–50 mL/min	GFR <10 mL/min	
Angiotensin-Converting Enzyme Inhibitors						
Benazepril	10 mg every day	20%	100%	75%	25%–50%	Hyperkalemia, acute renal failure, angioedema, rash, cough, anemia, and liver toxicity
Captopril	6.25–25 mg by mouth 3 times a day	35%	100%	75%	50%	Rare proteinuria, nephrotic syndrome, dysgeusia, granulocytopenia. Increases serum digoxin levels
Enalapril	5 mg every day	45%	100%	75%	50%	Enalaprilat, the active moiety formed in liver
Fosinopril	10 mg by mouth every day	20%	100%	100%	75%	Fosinoprilat, the active moiety formed in liver. Drug less likely than other angiotensin-converting enzyme inhibitors to accumulate in renal failure
Lisinopril	2.5 mg every day	80%	100%	50%–75%	25%–50%	Lysine analogue of a pharmacologically active enalapril metabolite

(continued on next page)

Table 5
(continued)

Antihypertensive and Cardiovascular Agents	Normal Dosage	% of Renal Excretion	Dosage Adjustment in Renal Failure			Comments
			GFR >50 mL/min	GFR 10–50 mL/min	GFR <10 mL/min	
Pentopril	125 mg every 24 h	80%–90%	100%	50%–75%	50%	
Perindopril	2 mg every 24 h	<10%	100%	75%	50%	Active metabolite is perindoprilat. The clearance of perindoprilat and its metabolites is almost exclusively renal. Approximately 60% of circulating perindopril is bound to plasma proteins, and only 10%–20% of perindoprilat is bound
Quinapril	10 mg every day / 20 mg every day	30%	100%	75%–100%	75%	Active metabolite is quinaprilat. 96% of quinaprilat is excreted renally
Ramipril	2.5 mg every day / 10 2 times a day	15%	100%	50%–75%	25%–50%	Active metabolite is ramiprilat. Data are for ramiprilat
Trandolapril	1–2 mg every day / 4 mg every day	33%	100%	50%–100%	50%	
Angiotensin-II Receptor Antagonists						Hyperkalemia, angioedema (less common than angiotensin-converting enzyme inhibitors)

Candesartan	16 mg every day	32 mg every day	33%	100%	100%	50%	Candesartan cilexetil is rapidly and completely bioactivated by ester hydrolysis during absorption from the gastrointestinal tract to candesartan
Eprosartan	600 mg every day	400–800 mg every day	25%	100%	100%	100%	Eprosartan pharmacokinetics more variable ESRD. Decreased protein binding in uremia
Irbesartan	150 mg every day	300 mg every day	20%	100%	100%	100%	
Losartan	50 mg every day	100 mg every day	13%	100%	100%	100%	
Valsartan	80 mg every day	160 mg 2 times a day	7%	100%	100%	100%	
Telmisartan	20–80 mg every day		<5%	100%	100%	100%	
β-Blockers							Decrease high-density lipoprotein, mask symptoms of hypoglycemia, bronchospasm, fatigue, insomnia, depression, and sexual dysfunction
Acebutolol	400 mg every 24 h or 2 times a day	600 mg every 24 h or 2 times a day	55%	100%	50%	30%–50%	Active metabolites with long half-life

(continued on next page)

Table 5
(continued)

Antihypertensive and Cardiovascular Agents	Normal Dosage		% of Renal Excretion	Dosage Adjustment in Renal Failure			Comments
				GFR >50 mL/min	GFR 10–50 mL/min	GFR <10 mL/min	
Atenolol	25 mg every day	100 mg every day	90%	100%	75%	50%	Accumulates in ESRD
Betaxolol	20 mg every 24 h	80%–90%	100%	100%	50%	50%	
Bopindolol	1 mg every 24 h	4 mg every 24 h	<10%	100%	100%	100%	
Carteolol	0.5 mg every 24 h	10 mg every 24 h	<50%	100%	50%	25%	
Carvedilol	3.125 mg by mouth 3 times a day	25 mg 3 times a day	2%	100%	100%	100%	Kinetics are dose dependent. Plasma concentrations of carvedilol have been reported to be increased in patients with renal impairment
Celiprolol	200 mg every 24 h		10%	100%	100%	75%	
Dilevalol	200 mg 2 times a day	400 mg 2 times a day	<5%	100%	100%	100%	
Esmolol (intravenously only)	50 µg/kg/min	300 µg/kg/min	10%	100%	100%	100%	Active metabolite retained in renal failure

Drug							Comments
Labetalol	50 mg by mouth 2 times a day	400 mg 2 times a day	5%	100%	100%	100%	For intravenous use: 20 mg slow intravenous injection over a 2-min period. Additional injections of 40 mg or 80 mg can be given at 10-min intervals until a total of 300 mg or continuous infusion of 2 mg/min
Metoprolol	50 mg 2 times a day	100 mg 2 times a day	<5%	100%	100%	100%	
Nadolol	80 mg every day	160 mg 2 times a day	90%	100%	50%	25%	Start with prolonged interval and titrate
Penbutolol	10 mg every 24 h	40 mg every 24 h	<10%	100%	100%	100%	
Pindolol	10 mg 2 times a day	40 mg 2 times a day	40%	100%	100%	100%	
Propranolol	40–160 mg 3 times a day	320 mg/d	<5%	100%	100%	100%	Bioavailability may increase in ESRD. Metabolites may cause increased bilirubin by assay interference in ESRD. Hypoglycemia reported in ESRD

(continued on next page)

Table 5
(continued)

Antihypertensive and Cardiovascular Agents	Normal Dosage	% of Renal Excretion	Dosage Adjustment in Renal Failure			Comments
			GFR >50 mL/min	GFR 10–50 mL/min	GFR <10 mL/min	
Sotalol	80 2 times a day	160 mg 2 times a day	70%	100%	50%	25%–50%	Extreme caution should be exercised in the use of sotalol in patients with renal failure undergoing hemodialysis. To minimize the risk of induced arrhythmia, patients initiated or reinitiated on BETAPACE should be placed for a minimum of 3 d (on their maintenance dose) in a facility that can provide cardiac resuscitation and continuous electrocardiographic monitoring
Timolol	10 mg 2 times a day	20 mg 2 times a day	15%	100%	100%	100%	

Calcium Channel Blockers

Dihydropyridine: headache, ankle edema, gingival hyperplasia and flushing
Nondihydropyridine: bradycardia, constipation, gingival hyperplasia and arteriovenous block

Drug	Dose	Dose	%	%	%	Comments
Amlodipine	2.5 by mouth every day	10 mg every day	10%	100%	100%	100%	May increase digoxin and cyclosporine levels
Bepridil	No data	<1%	No data	No data	No data		Weak vasodilator and antihypertensive.
Diltiazem	30 mg 3 times a day	90 mg 3 times a day	10%	100%	100%	100%	Acute renal dysfunction. May exacerbate hyperkalemia. May increase digoxin and cyclosporine levels
Felodipine	5 mg by mouth 2 times a day	20 mg every day	1%	100%	100%	100%	May increase digoxin levels
Isradipine	5 mg by mouth 2 times a day	10 mg 2 times a day	<5%	100%	100%	100%	May increase digoxin levels
Nicardipine	20 mg by mouth 3 times a day	30 mg by mouth 3 times a day	<1%	100%	100%	100%	Uremia inhibits hepatic metabolism. May increase digoxin levels
Nifedipine XL	30 every day	90 mg 2 times a day	10%	100%	100%	100%	Avoid short-acting nifedipine formulation

(continued on next page)

Table 5
(continued)

| Antihypertensive and Cardiovascular Agents | Normal Dosage | % of Renal Excretion | Dosage Adjustment in Renal Failure | | | Comments |
			GFR >50 mL/min	GFR 10–50 mL/min	GFR <10 mL/min	
Nimodipine	30 mg every 8 h	10%	100%	100%	100%	May lower blood pressure
Nisoldipine	20 mg every day	10%	100%	100%	100%	May increase digoxin levels
Verapamil	40 mg 3 times a day	10%	100%	100%	100%	Acute renal dysfunction. Active metabolites accumulate particularly with sustained-release forms
Diuretics						Hypokalemia/hyperkalemia (potassium-sparing agents), hyperuricemia, hyperglycemia, hypomagnesemia, increase serum cholesterol
Acetazolamide	125 mg by mouth 3 times a day	90%	100%	50%	Avoid	May potentiate acidosis. Ineffective as diuretic in ESRD. May cause neurologic side effects in dialysis patients

Acetazolamide alternate dosage: 500 mg by mouth 3 times a day

Drug	Dose						Comments
Amiloride	5 mg by mouth every day	10 mg by mouth every day	50%	100%	100%	Avoid	Hyperkalemia with GFR <30 mL/min, especially in diabetics. Hyperchloremic metabolic acidosis
Bumetanide	1–2 mg by mouth every day	2–4 mg by mouth every day	35%	100%	100%	100%	Ototoxicity increased in ESRD in combination with aminoglycosides. High doses effective in ESRD. Muscle pain, gynecomastia
Chlorthalidone	25 mg every 24 h	50%	Every 24 h	Every 24 h	Avoid	Ineffective with low GFR	
Ethacrynic acid	50 mg by mouth every day	100 mg by mouth 2 times a day	20%	100%	100%	100%	Ototoxicity increased in ESRD in combination with aminoglycosides
Furosemide	40–80 mg by mouth every day	120 mg by mouth 3 times a day	70%	100%	100%	100%	Ototoxicity increased in ESRD, especially in combination with aminoglycosides. High doses effective in ESRD
Indapamide	2.5 mg every 24 h	<5%	100%	100%	Avoid	Ineffective in ESRD	
Metolazone	2.5 mg by mouth every day	10 mg by mouth 2 times a day	70%	100%	100%		High doses effective in ESRD. Gynecomastia, impotence
Piretanide	6 mg every 24 h	12 mg every 24 h	40%–60%	100%	100%	100%	High doses effective in ESRD. Ototoxicity

(continued on next page)

Table 5
(continued)

Antihypertensive and Cardiovascular Agents	Normal Dosage		% of Renal Excretion	Dosage Adjustment in Renal Failure			Comments
				GFR >50 mL/min	GFR 10–50 mL/min	GFR <10 mL/min	
Spironolactone	100 mg by mouth every day	300 mg by mouth every day	25%	100%	100%	Avoid	Active metabolites with long half-life. Hyperkalemia common when GFR <30 mL/min, especially in diabetics. Gynecomastia, hyperchloremic acidosis. Increases serum by immunoassay interference
Thiazides	25 mg 2 times a day	50 mg 2 times a day		>95%	100%	100%	Avoid
Torasemide	5 mg by mouth 2 times a day	20 mg every day	25%	100%	100%	100%	High doses effective in ESRD. Ototoxicity
Triamterene	25 mg 2 times a day	50 mg 2 times a day	5%–10%	Every 12 h	Every 12 h	Avoid	Hyperkalemia common when GFR <30 mL/min, especially in diabetics. Active metabolite with long half-life in ESRD. Folic acid antagonist. Urolithiasis. Crystalluria in acid urine. May cause acute renal failure

Miscellaneous Agents

Drug							Toxicity/Notes
Amrinone	5 mg/kg/min daily dose <10 mg/kg	10 mg/kg/min daily does <10 mg/kg	10%–40%	100%	100%	100%	Thrombocytopenia. Nausea, vomiting in ESRD
Clonidine	0.1 by mouth 2 times a day/3 times a day	1.2 mg/d	45%	100%	100%	100%	Sexual dysfunction, dizziness, postal hypotension
Digoxin	0.125 mg every other day/every day	0.25 mg by mouth every day	25%	100%	100%	100%	Decrease loading dose by 50% in ESRD. Radioimmunoassay may overestimate serum levels in uremia. Clearance decreased by amiodarone, spironolactone, quinidine, verapamil. Hypokalemia, hypomagnesemia enhance toxicity. Vd and total body clearance decreased in ESRD. Serum level 12 h after dose is best guide in ESRD. Digoxin immune antibodies can treat severe toxicity in ESRD
Hydralazine	10 mg by mouth 4 times a day	100 mg by mouth 4 times a day	25%	100%	100%	100%	Lupuslike reaction
Midodrine	No data	No data	75%–80%	5–10 mg every 8 h	5–10 mg every 8 h	No data	Increased blood pressure

(continued on next page)

Table 5
(continued)

Antihypertensive and Cardiovascular Agents	Normal Dosage		% of Renal Excretion	Dosage Adjustment in Renal Failure			Comments
				GFR >50 mL/min	GFR 10–50 mL/min	GFR <10 mL/min	
Minoxidil	2.5 mg by mouth 2 times a day	10 mg by mouth 2 times a day	20%	100%	100%	100%	Pericardial effusion, fluid retention, hypertrichosis, and tachycardia
Nitroprusside	1 µg/kg/min	10 µg/kg/min	<10%	100%	100%	100%	Cyanide toxicity
Amrinone	5 µg/kg/min	10 µg/kg/min	25%	100%	100%	100%	Thrombocytopenia. Nausea, vomiting in ESRD
Dobutamine	2.5 µg/kg/min	15 µg/kg/min	10%	100%	100%	100%	
Milrinone	0.375 µg/kg/min	0.75 µg/kg/min		100%	100%	100%	

Table 6
Endocrine and metabolic agent dosing in renal failure

Hypoglycemic Agents	Normal Dosage	% of Renal Excretion	Dosage Adjustment in Renal Failure			Comments
			GFR >50 mL/min	GFR 10–50 mL/min	GFR <10 mL/min	
Acarbose	25 mg 3 times a day	35%	100%	50%	Avoid	Avoid all oral hypoglycemic agents on continuous renal replacement therapy. Abdominal pain, nausea/vomiting, and flatulence
Acetohexamide	250 mg every 24 h	None	Avoid	Avoid	Avoid	Diuretic effect. May falsely increase serum creatinine. Active metabolite has $T_{1/2}$ of 5–8 h in healthy individuals and is eliminated by the kidney. Prolonged hypoglycemia in azotemic patients
Chlorpropamide	100 mg every 24 h	47%	50%	Avoid	Avoid	Impairs water excretion. Prolonged hypoglycemia in azotemic patients
Glibornuride	12.5 mg every 14 h	No data	No data	No data	No data	

(continued on next page)

Table 6
(continued)

Hypoglycemic Agents	Normal Dosage	% of Renal Excretion	Dosage Adjustment in Renal Failure			Comments
			GFR >50 mL/min	GFR 10–50 mL/min	GFR <10 mL/min	
Gliclazide	80 mg every 24 h	320 mg every 24 h	<20%	50%–100%	Avoid	Avoid	
Glipizide	5 mg every day	20 mg 2 times a day	5%	100%	50%	50%	
Glyburide	2.5 mg every day	10 mg 2 times a day	50%	100%	50%	Avoid	
Metformin	500 mg 2 times a day	2550 mg/d (2 times a day or 3 times a day)	95%	100%	Avoid	Avoid	Lactic acidosis
Repaglinide	0.5–1 mg	4 mg 3 times a day					
Tolazamide	100 mg every 24 h	250 mg every 24 h	7%	100%	100%	100%	Diuretic effects
Tolbutamide	1 g every 24 h	2 g every 24 h	None	100%	100%	100%	May impair water excretion
Troglitazone	200 mg every day	600 mg every day	3%	100%	Avoid	Avoid	Decreases cyclosporine A level, Hepatotoxic
Parenteral Agents							Dosage guided by blood glucose levels
Insulin	Variable		None	100%	75%	50%	Renal metabolism of insulin decreases with azotemia
Lispro insulin	Variable		No data	100%	75%	50%	Avoid all oral hypoglycemic agents on continuous renal replacement therapy

Table 7
Endocrine and metabolic agent dosing in renal failure

Hyperlipidemic Agents	Normal Dosage	% of Renal Excretion	Dosage Adjustment in Renal Failure			Comments
			GFR >50 mL/min	GFR 10–50 mL/min	GFR <10 mL/min	
Atorvastatin	10 mg/d	<2%	100%	100%	100%	Liver dysfunction, myalgia and rhabdomyolysis with CSA/FK
	80 mg/d					
Bezafibrate	200 mg 2 times a day–4 times a day 400 mg SR every 24 h	50%	50%–100%	25%–50%	Avoid	
Cholestyramine	4 g 2 times a day	None	100%	100%	100%	
Clofibrate	500 mg 2 times a day 1000 mg 2 times a day	40%–70%	Every 6–12 h	Every 12–18 h	Avoid	
Colestipol	5 g 2 times a day	None	100%	100%	100%	
Fluvastatin	20 mg daily 80 mg/d	<1%	100%	100%	100%	
Gemfibrozil	600 mg 2 times a day 600 mg 2 times a day	None	100%	100%	100%	
Lovastatin	5 mg daily 20 mg/d	None	100%	100%	100%	
Nicotinic acid	1 g 3 times a day 2 g 3 times a day	None	100%	50%	25%	
Pravastatin	10–40 mg daily 80 mg daily	<10%	100%	100%	100%	
Probucol	500 mg 2 times a day	<2%	100%	100%	100%	
Crestor	5–20 mg/d 40 mg/d		100%	100%	100%	
Simvastatin	5–20 mg daily 20 mg/d	13%	100%	100%	100%	

Table 8
Antithyroid dosing in renal failure

Antithyroid Drugs	Normal Dosage	% of Renal Excretion	Dosage Adjustment in Renal Failure			Comments
			GFR >50 mL/min	GFR 10–50 mL/min	GFR <10 mL/min	
Methimazole	5–20 mg 3 times a day	7%	100%	100%	100%	
Propylthiouracil	100 mg 3 times a day	<10%	100%	100%	100%	

Step 5: Drug Level Monitoring

Therapeutic drug monitoring (TDM), although important in all ages, is essential in the elderly for medications with a narrow therapeutic index. The combination of comorbid conditions and age-related changes in pharmacokinetics and pharmacodynamics puts older adults at increased risk of toxicity. More precise estimates of renal function in the elderly and preemptive dosage changes can prevent adverse effects from over-exposure to drugs in the elderly. Assessment of drug levels allows for more careful monitoring of these medications. Appropriate dosing based on drug levels relies on accurate assessment of the timing of the level combined with the dose and route of administration of the drug being administered. Often drug levels are expensive and should not be used for dosing unless those levels have been established with toxicity or efficacy. Few drugs rely on peak levels for efficacy. On the other hand, trough levels are often used to assess drug level and efficacy in the body. They may be measured to ensure drug clearance despite potential reductions in excretion or metabolism that can occur in the elderly. Despite appropriate drug levels, patients must still be monitored closely for potential adverse effects that may be unrelated to the actual levels of drug in the body. For example, aminoglycosides such as gentamicin or tobramycin may have appropriate levels but can accumulate in the inner ear and renal tubules causing severe damage. Elderly patients and those with ESRD may have significant changes in protein binding of medications. For medications that are highly protein bound, drug assays of plasma concentration may be within therapeutic range while the patient is exhibiting sign of toxicity. The phenomenon occurs because of an increase in unbound drug exerting action within the body. Medications such as phenytoin may be assessed by free fraction in elderly patients with kidney disease. **Tables 1–15** provide TDM parameters in renal insufficiency for drugs for which routine monitoring is recommended.

SUMMARY

As the elderly population in the United States increases, health care professionals need to be aware of potential age-related changes that affect medication prescribing. Increased emphasis on careful patient assessment and safety can reduce the incidence of adverse events related to medications.

Table 9
Gastrointestinal agents

Gastrointestinal Agents	Normal Doses Starting Dose	Normal Doses Maximum Dose	% of Renal Excretion	Dosage Adjustment in Renal Failure GFR >50 mL/min	GFR 10–50 mL/min	GFR <10 mL/min	Comments
Cimetidine	300 mg by mouth 3 times a day	800 mg by mouth 2 times a day	60%	100%	75%	25%	Multiple drug-drug interactions: β-blockers, sulfonylurea, theophylline, warfarin, and so forth
Famotidine	20 mg by mouth 2 times a day	40 mg by mouth 2 times a day	70%	100%	75%	25%	Headache, fatigue, thrombocytopenia, alopecia
Lansoprazole	15 mg by mouth every day	30 mg 2 times a day	None	100%	100%	100%	Headache, diarrhea
Nizatidine	150 mg by mouth 2 times a day	300 mg by mouth 2 times a day	20%	100%	75%	25%	Headache, fatigue, thrombocytopenia, alopecia
Omeprazole	20 mg by mouth every day	40 mg by mouth 2 times a day	None	100%	100%	100%	Headache, diarrhea
Rabeprazole	20 mg by mouth every day	40 mg by mouth 2 times a day	None	100%	100%	100%	Headache, diarrhea
Pantoprazole	40 mg by mouth every day	80 mg by mouth 2 times a day	None	100%	100%	100%	Headache, diarrhea
Ranitidine	150 mg by mouth 2 times a day	300 mg by mouth 2 times a day	80%	100%	75%	25%	Headache, fatigue, thrombocytopenia, alopecia
Cisapride	10 mg by mouth 3 times a day	20 mg 4 times a day	5%	100%	100%	50%–75%	Avoid with azole antifungal, macrolide antibiotics, and other P450 IIIA-4 inhibitors
Metoclopramide	10 mg by mouth 3 times a day	30 mg by mouth 4 times a day	15%	100%	100%	50%–75%	Increase cyclosporine/tacrolimus level. Neurotoxic
Misoprostol	100 µg by mouth 2 times a day	200 µg by mouth 4 times a day	100%	100%	100%	100%	Diarrhea, nausea/vomiting Abortifacient agent
Sucralfate	1 g by mouth 4 times a day	1 g by mouth 4 times a day	None	100%	100%	100%	Constipation, decrease absorption of mycophenolate mofetil

Table 10
Neurologic/anticonvulsant dosing in renal failure

Anticonvulsants	Normal Dosage	% of Renal Excretion	Dosage Adjustment in Renal Failure			Comments
			GFR >50 mL/min	GFR 10–50 mL/min	GFR <10 mL/min	
Carbamazepine	2–8 mg/kg/d, adjust for side effects and TDM	2%	100%	100%	100%	Plasma concentration: 4–12 mcg/ml, double vision, fluid retention, mylosuppression
Clonazepam	0.5 mg 3 times a day	1%	100%	100%	100%	Although no dose reduction is recommended, the drug has not been studied in patients with renal impairment. Recommendations are based on known drug characteristics not clinical trials data
Ethosuximide	5 mg/kg/d, adjust for side effects and TDM	20%	100%	100%	100%	Plasma concentration: 40–100 mcg/ml, headache
Felbamate	1200 mg/3 times a day	90%	100%	50%	25%	Anorexia, vomiting, insomnia, nausea
Gabapentin	900 mg 3 times a day	77%	100%	50%	25%	Less central nervous system side effects compared with other agents
Lamotrigine	150 mg/d	1%	100%	100%	100%	Autoinduction, major drug-drug interaction with valproate
Levetiracetam	500 mg 2 times a day	66%	100%	50%	50%	
Oxcarbazepine	300 mg 2 times a day	1%	100%	100%	100%	Less effect on P450 compared with carbamazepine
Phenobarbital	20 mg/kg/d, adjust for side effects and TDM	1%	100%	100%	100%	Plasma concentration: 15–40 mcg/ml, insomnia

Drug	Dose		Adjust for renal failure and low Albumin			Comments
Phenytoin	20 mg/kg/d, adjust for side effects and TDM	1%				Plasma concentration: 10–20, nystagmus, check free phenytoin level
Primidone	50 mg	1%	100%	100%	100%	Plasma concentration: 5–20
Sodium valproate	7.5–15 mg/kg/d, adjust for side effects and TDM	1%	100%	100%	100%	Plasma concentration: 50–150, weight gain, hepatitis, check free valproate level
Tiagabine	4 mg every day, increase 4 mg/d, titrate weekly	2%	100%	100%	100%	Total daily dose may be increased by 4–8 mg at weekly intervals until clinical response is achieved or up to 32 mg/d. The total daily dose should be given in divided doses 2 to 4 times daily
Topiramate	50 mg/d	70%	100%	50%	Avoid	Kidney stone
Trimethadione	300 mg 3–4 times a day	None	Every 8 h	Every 8–12 h	Every 12–24 h	Active metabolites with long half-life in ESRD. Nephrotic syndrome
Vigabatrin	1 g 2 times a day	70%	100%	50%	25%	Encephalopathy with drug accumulation
Zonisamide	100–300 mg every day, 2 times a day	30%	100%	75%	50%	Manufacturer recommends that zonisamide should not be used in patients with renal failure (estimated GFR <50 mL/min) as there has been insufficient experience concerning drug dosing and toxicity. Zonisamide doses of 100–600 mg/d are effective for normal renal function. Dose recommendations for renal impairment based on clearance ratios

Table 11
Rheumatologic dosing in renal failure

Arthritis and Gout Agents	Normal Dosage	% of Renal Excretion	GFR >50 mL/min	GFR 10–50 mL/min	GFR <10 mL/min	Comments
Allopurinol	300 mg every 24 h	30%	75%	50%	25%	Interstitial nephritis. Rare xanthine stones. Renal excretion of active metabolite with $T_{1/2}$ of 25 h in normal renal function- $T_{1/2}$ 1 wk in patients with ESRD. Exfoliative dermatitis
Auranofin	6 mg every 24 h	50%	50%	Avoid	Avoid	Proteinuria and nephritic syndrome
Colchicine	Acute: 2 mg then 0.5 mg every 6 h Chronic: 0.5–1.0 mg every 24 h	5%–17%	100%	50%–100%	25%	Avoid prolonged use if GFR <50 mL/min
Gold sodium	25–50 mg	60%–90%	50%	Avoid	Avoid	Thiomalate proteinuria, nephritic syndrome, membranous nephritis
Penicillamine	250–1000 mg every 24 h	40%	100%	Avoid	Avoid	Nephrotic syndrome
Probenecid	500 mg 2 times a day	<2%	100%	Avoid	Avoid	Ineffective at decreased GFR
Nonsteroidal Antiinflammatory Drugs						May decrease renal function. Decrease platelet aggregation. Nephrotic syndrome. Interstitial nephritis. Hyperkalemia. Sodium retention
Diclofenac	25–75 mg 2 times a day	<1%	50%–100%	25%–50%	25%	
Diflunisal	250–500 mg 2 times a day	<3%	100%	50%	50%	

Dosage Adjustment in Renal Failure

Etodolac	200 mg 2 times a day	Negligible	100%	100%	100%	
Fenoprofen	300–600 mg 4 times a day	30%	100%	100%	100%	
Flurbiprofen	100 mg 2 to 3 times a day	20%	100%	100%	100%	
Ibuprofen	800 mg 3 times a day	1%	100%	100%	100%	
Indomethacin	25–50 mg 3 times a day	30%	100%	100%	100%	
Ketoprofen	25–75 mg 3 times a day	<1%	100%	100%	100%	
Ketorolac	30–60 mg load then 15–30 mg every 6 h	30%–60%	100%	50%	25%–50%	Acute hearing loss in ESRD
Meclofenamic acid	50–100 mg 3–4 times a day	2%–4%	100%	100%	100%	
Mefanamic acid	250 mg 4 times a day	<6%	100%	100%	100%	
Nabumetone	1.0–2.0 g every 24 h	<1%	100%	50%–100%	50%–100%	
Naproxen	500 mg 2 times a day	<1%	100%	100%	100%	
Oxaproxin	1200 mg every 24 h	<1%	100%	100%	100%	
Phenylbutazone	100 mg 3–4 times a day	1%	100%	100%	100%	
Piroxicam	20 mg every 24 h	10%	100%	100%	100%	
Sulindac	200 mg 2 times a day	7%	100%	100%	100%	Active sulfide metabolite in ESRD
Tolmetin	400 mg 3 times a day	15%	100%	100%	100%	

Table 12
Sedative dosing in renal failure

Sedatives	Normal Dosage	% of Renal Excretion	Dosage Adjustment in Renal Failure GFR >50 mL/min	GFR 10–50 mL/min	GFR <10 mL/min	Comments
Barbiturates						
Pentobarbital	30 mg every 6–8 h	Hepatic	100%	100%	100%	May cause excessive sedation, increase osteomalacia in ESRD. Charcoal hemoperfusion and hemodialysis more effective than peritoneal dialysis for poisoning
Phenobarbital	50–100 mg every 8–12 h	Hepatic (renal)	Every 8–12 h	Every 8–12 h	Every 12–16 h	Up to 50% unchanged drug excreted with urine with alkaline diuresis
Secobarbital	30–50 mg every 6–8 h	Hepatic	100%	100%	100%	
Thiopental	Anesthesia induction (individualized)	Hepatic	100%	100%	100%	
Benzodiazepines						May cause excessive sedation and encephalopathy in ESRD
Alprazolam	0.25–5.0 mg every 8 h	Hepatic	100%	100%	100%	
Clorazepate	15–60 mg every 24 h	Hepatic (renal)	100%	100%	100%	
Chlordiazepoxide	15–100 mg every 24 h	Hepatic	100%	100%	50%	
Clonazepam	1.5 mg every 24 h	Hepatic	100%	100%	100%	Although no dose reduction is recommended, the drug has not been studied in patients with renal impairment. Recommendations are based on known drug characteristics not clinical trials data
Diazepam	5–40 mg every 24 h	Hepatic	100%	100%	100%	Active metabolites, desmethyldiazepam and oxazepam may accumulate in renal failure. Dose should be reduced if given longer than a few days. Protein binding decreases in uremia
Estazolam	1 mg every h	Hepatic	100%	100%	100%	

Flurazepam	15–30 mg every h	Hepatic	100%	100%	100%	
Lorazepam	1–2 mg every 8–12 h	Hepatic	100%	100%	100%	
Midazolam	Individualized	Hepatic	100%	100%	50%	
Oxazepam	30–120 mg every 24 h	Hepatic	100%	100%	100%	
Quazepam	15 mg every h	Hepatic	No data	No data	No data	
Temazepam	30 mg every h	Hepatic	100%	100%	100%	
Triazolam	0.25–0.50 mg every h	Hepatic	100%	100%	100%	Protein binding correlates with α-1 acid glycoprotein concentration
Benzodiazepine Antagonist						May cause excessive sedation and encephalopathy in ESRD
Flumazenil	0.2 mg intravenously over 15 s	Hepatic	100%	100%	100%	
Miscellaneous Sedative Agents						
Buspirone	5 mg every 8 h	Hepatic	100%	100%	100%	
Ethchlorvynol	500 mg every h	Hepatic	100%	Avoid	Avoid	Removed by hemoperfusion. Excessive sedation
Haloperidol	1–2 mg every 8–12 h	Hepatic	100%	100%	100%	Hypertension, excessive sedation
Lithium carbonate	0.9–1.2 g every 24 h	Renal	100%	50%–75%	25%–50%	Nephrotoxic. Nephrogenic diabetes insipidus. Nephrotic syndrome. Renal tubular acidosis. Interstitial fibrosis. Acute toxicity when serum levels >1.2 mEq/L. Serum levels should be measure periodically 12 h after dose. $T_{1/2}$ does not reflect extensive tissue accumulation. Plasma levels rebound after dialysis. Toxicity enhanced by volume depletion, nonsteroidal antiinflammatory drugs, and diuretics
Meprobamate	1.2–1.6 g every 24 h	Hepatic (renal)	Every 6 h	Every 9–12 h	Every 12–18 h	Excessive sedation. Excretion enhanced by forced diuresis

Table 13
Anti-Parkinson dosing in renal failure

Anti-Parkinson Agents	Normal Dosage	% of Renal Excretion	Dosage Adjustment in Renal Failure			Comments
			GFR >50 mL/min	GFR 10–50 mL/min	GFR <10 mL/min	
Carbidopa	1 tablet 3 times a day to 6 tablets daily	30%	100%	100%	100%	Require careful titration of dose according to clinical response
Levodopa	25–500 mg 2 times a day to 8 g every 24 h	None	100%	50%– 100%	50%– 100%	Active and inactive metabolites excreted in urine. Active metabolites with long $T_{1/2}$ in ESRD

Table 14
Antipsychotic dosing in renal failure

Antipsychotics	Normal Dosage	% of Renal Excretion	Dosage Adjustment in Renal Failure			Comments
			GFR >50 mL/min	GFR 10–50 mL/min	GFR <10 mL/min	
Phenothiazines						
Chlorpromazine	300–800 mg every 24 h	Hepatic	100%	100%	100%	Orthostatic hypotension, extrapyramidal symptoms, and confusion can occur
Promethazine	20–100 mg every 24 h	Hepatic	100%	100%	100%	No comments
Thioridazine	50–100 mg by mouth 3 times a day. Increase gradually. Maximum of 800 mg/d	Hepatic	100%	100%	100%	Excessive sedation may occur in ESRD
Trifluoperazine	1–2 mg 2 times a day. Increase to no more than 6 mg	Hepatic	100%	100%	100%	
Perphenazine	8–16 mg by mouth 2, 3, or 4 times a day. Increase to 64 mg daily	Hepatic	100%	100%	100%	
Thiothixene	2 mg by mouth 3 times a day. Increase gradually to 15 mg daily	Hepatic	100%	100%	100%	
Haloperidol	1–2 mg every 8–12 h	Hepatic	100%	100%	100%	Hypotension, excessive sedation
Loxapine	12.5–50 mg intramuscularly every 4–6 h					Do not administer drug intravenously
Clozapine	12.5 mg by mouth. 25–50 mg daily to 300–450 mg by end of 2 wk. Maximum: 900 mg daily	Metabolism nearly complete	100%	100%	100%	
Risperidone	1 mg by mouth 2 times a day. Increase to 3 mg 2 times a day		100%	100%	100%	
Olanzapine	5–10 mg	Hepatic	100%	100%	100%	Potential hypotensive effects
Quetiapine	25 mg by mouth 2 times a day. Increase in increments of 25–50 mg 2 or 3 times a day. 300–400 mg daily by day 4	Hepatic	100%	100%	100%	
Ziprasideone	20–100 mg every 12 h	Hepatic	100%	100%	100%	

Table 15
Miscellaneous dosing in renal failure

Drug	Normal Dosage	% of Renal Excretion	Dosage Adjustment in Renal Failure			Comments
			GFR >50 mL/min	GFR 10–50 mL/min	GFR <10 mL/min	
Corticosteroids						May aggravate azotemia, Na$^+$ retention, glucose intolerance, and hypertension
Betamethasone	0.5–9.0 mg every 24 h	5	100%	100%	100%	
Budesonide	No data	None	100%	100%	100%	
Cortisone	25–500 mg every 24 h	None	100%	100%	100%	
Dexamethasone	0.75–9.0 mg every 24 h	8	100%	100%	100%	
Hydrocortisone	20–500 mg every 24 h	None	100%	100%	100%	
Methylprednisolone	4–48 mg every 24 h	<10	100%	100%	100%	
Prednisolone	5–60 mg every 24 h	34	100%	100%	100%	
Prednisone	5–60 mg every 24 h	34	100%	100%	100%	
Triamcinolone	4–48 mg every 24 h	No data	100%	100%	100%	
Anticoagulants						
Alteplase	60 mg over 1 h then 20 mg/h for 2 h	No data	100%	100%	100%	Tissue-type plasminogen activator
Aspirin	325 mg/d 81 mg/d	10%	100%	100%	100%	Gastrointestinal irritation and bleeding tendency
Clopidogrel	75 mg/d	50%	100%	100%	100%	Gastrointestinal irritation and bleeding tendency
Dalteparin	2500 units subcutaneously/d 5000 units subcutaneously/d	Unknown	100%	100%	50%	

Drug	Dose					Comments
Dipyridamole	50 mg 3 times a day	No data	100%	100%	100%	
Enoxaparin	20 mg/d	8%	100%	75%–50%	50%	1 mg/kg every 12 h for treatment of deep vein thrombosis. Check antifactor Xa activity 4 h after second dose in patients with renal dysfunction. Some evidence of drug accumulation in renal failure
	30 mg 2 times a day					
Heparin	75 U/kg load then 15 U/kg/h	None	100%	100%	100%	Half-life increases with dose
Iloprost	0.5–2.0 ng/kg/min for 5–12 h	No data	100%	100%	50%	
Indobufen	100 mg 2 times a day	<15%	100%	50%	50%	
	200 mg 2 times a day					
Streptokinase	250,000 U/kg load then 100,000 U/h	None	100%	50%	25%	
Sulfinpyrazone	200 mg 2 times a day	25%–50%	100%	100%	100%	Acute renal failure. Uricosuric effect at low GFR
Ticlopidine	250 mg 2 times a day	2%	100%	100%	Avoid	Decrease cyclosporine A level, may cause severe neutropenia and thrombocytopenia
	250 mg 2 times a day					
Tranexamic acid	25 mg/kg 3–4 times a day	90%	50%	25%	10%	
Urokinase	4400 U/kg load then 4400 U/kg every hour	No data	No data	No data	No data	
Warfarin	2.5–5 mg/d	<1%	100%	100%	100%	Monitor international normalized ratio closely. Start at 5 mg/d. 1 mg vitamin K intravenously over 30 min or 2.5–5 mg by mouth can be used to normalize international normalized ratio
	Adjust per international normalized ratio					

REFERENCES

1. Available at: www.aoa.gov/aoaroot/...statistics/.../By_Age_65_and_over.xls. Accessed March 2013.
2. Available at: http://www.agingstats.gov/Main_Site/Data/2012_Documents/Health_Care.aspx. Accessed March 2013.
3. Miller SW. Evaluating medication regimens in the elderly. Consult Pharm 2008; 23(7):538–47.
4. Sitar DS. Aging issues in drug disposition and efficacy. Proc West Pharmacol Soc 2007;50:16–20.
5. Aronow WS. Treatment of hypertension in the elderly. Compr Ther 2008;34(3–4): 171–6.
6. Gray SL, Lai KV, Larson EB. Drug-induced cognition disorders in the elderly: incidence, prevention and management. Drug Saf 1999;21(2):101–22.
7. Levy RH, Collins C. Risk and predictability of drug interactions in the elderly. Int Rev Neurobiol 2007;81:235–51.
8. Muhlberg W, Platt D. Age-dependent changes of the kidneys: pharmacological implications. Gerontology 1999;45(5):243–53.
9. Lindeman RD, Tobin J, Shock NW. Longitudinal studies on the rate of decline in renal function with age. J Am Geriatr Soc 1985;33(4):278–85.
10. ElDesoky ES. Pharmacokinetic-pharmacodynamic crisis in the elderly. Am J Ther 2007;14(5):488–98.
11. Olyaei AJ, Bennett WM. Drug dosing in the elderly patients with chronic kidney disease. Clin Geriatr Med 2009;25(3):459–527.
12. Barnett SR. Polypharmacy and perioperative medications in the elderly. Anesthesiol Clin 2009;27(3):377–89 table.
13. Chau DL, Walker V, Pai L, et al. Opiates and elderly: use and side effects. Clin Interv Aging 2008;3(2):273–8.
14. McLean AJ, Le Couteur DG. Aging biology and geriatric clinical pharmacology. Pharmacol Rev 2004;56(2):163–84.
15. Ferrario CG. Geropharmacology: a primer for advanced practice acute care and critical care nurses, part I. AACN Adv Crit Care 2008;19(1):23–35.
16. Stevens LA, Padala S, Levey AS. Advances in glomerular filtration rate-estimating equations. Curr Opin Nephrol Hypertens 2010;19(3):298–307.
17. Cockcroft DW, Gault MH. Prediction of creatinine clearance from serum creatinine. Nephron 1976;16(1):31–41.
18. Levey AS, Stevens LA, Schmid CH, et al. A new equation to estimate glomerular filtration rate. Ann Intern Med 2009;150(9):604–12.
19. Levey AS, Stevens LA. Estimating GFR using the CKD Epidemiology Collaboration (CKD-EPI) creatinine equation: more accurate GFR estimates, lower CKD prevalence estimates, and better risk predictions. Am J Kidney Dis 2010;55(4): 622–7.
20. Stevens LA, Schmid CH, Greene T, et al. Comparative performance of the CKD Epidemiology Collaboration (CKD-EPI) and the Modification of Diet in Renal Disease (MDRD) study equations for estimating GFR levels above 60 mL/min/ 1.73 m². Am J Kidney Dis 2010;56(3):486–95.
21. Zhou XJ, Rakheja D, Yu X, et al. The aging kidney. Kidney Int 2008;74(6): 710–20.
22. Minaker KL. Common clinical sequelae of aging. In: Goldman L, Schafer AI, editors. Goldman's Cecil medicine. 24th edition. Philadelphia: Saunders Elsevier; 2012. Chapter 24.

23. Available at: http://www.cdc.gov/nchs/fastats/older_americans.htm. Accessed March 2013.
24. Flamant M, Haymann JP, Vidal-Petiot E, et al. GFR estimation using the Cockcroft-Gault, MDRD study, and CKD-EPI equations in the elderly. Am J Kidney Dis 2012; 60(5):847–9.
25. Available at: http://www.fda.gov/downloads/Drugs/.../Guidances/UCM204959. pdf. Accessed March 2013.
26. Stevens LA, Nolin TD, Richardson MM, et al. Comparison of drug dosing recommendations based on measured GFR and kidney function estimating equations. Am J Kidney Dis 2009;54(1):33–42.
27. Carter JL, Stevens PE, Irving JE, et al. Estimating glomerular filtration rate: comparison of the CKD-EPI and MDRD equations in a large UK cohort with particular emphasis on the effect of age. QJM 2011;104(10):839–47.
28. Olyaei AJ, Steffl JL. A quantitative approach to drug dosing in chronic kidney disease. Blood Purif 2011;31(1–3):138–45.
29. Levey AS, Coresh J, Greene T, et al. Using standardized serum creatinine values in the modification of diet in renal disease study equation for estimating glomerular filtration rate. Ann Intern Med 2006;145(4):247–54.
30. Levey AS, Bosch JP, Lewis JB, et al. A more accurate method to estimate glomerular filtration rate from serum creatinine: a new prediction equation. Modification of Diet in Renal Disease Study Group. Ann Intern Med 1999;130(6):461–70.

Transplantation in the Elderly Patient

Douglas Scott Keith, MD

KEYWORDS

- Kidney transplantation • Elderly • Immunosenescence • Immunosuppression
- Survival • Selection

KEY POINTS

- Whereas kidney transplantation is the treatment of choice for most young candidates due to its large survival advantage over dialysis, the risk benefit equation with regard to kidney transplantation is more complex in the geriatric candidate.
- Aging is associated with functional changes in the immune system and the accumulation of morbidity that affect the outcomes of kidney transplantation. For elderly candidates who are frail and have high levels of comorbidity, kidney transplantation may shorten life expectancy over continued dialysis. To date, however, among the highly selected population of geriatric kidney transplant recipients, both a quality of life and survival benefit over dialysis has been demonstrated.
- Properly selected geriatric candidates benefit from transplantation in many of the same ways as younger candidates. Unfortunately, due to increasing demand for kidneys and ever increasing waiting times, deceased donor kidney transplant as an option for the elderly is becoming more difficult due to their limited survival on dialysis.
- The organ shortage raises difficult questions regarding allocation of a scarce resource and how patients are selected for listing. There is no age limit for consideration of kidney transplantation, and the selection process remains largely subjective and at the whim of the transplant program.
- Given the growing geriatric end-stage renal disease population, not only is better research necessary to define those geriatric subgroups that benefit most from kidney transplantation but also is public discourse on how we allocate this scarce resource in an aging population.

INTRODUCTION

An increasing incidence of end-stage renal disease (ESRD) in the elderly and aging of the United States population have been the primary reason for continued growth of ESRD population.[1] The success of kidney transplantation as a treatment of ESRD has led to an increase in kidney transplantation in the elderly who were once thought

Disclosure: The author has no financial disclosures to make with regard to this article.
Department of Medicine, Division of Nephrology, University of Virginia Medical Center, PO Box 800133, Charlottesville, VA 22908-0133, USA
E-mail address: dsk9s@virginia.edu

Clin Geriatr Med 29 (2013) 707–719
http://dx.doi.org/10.1016/j.cger.2013.05.010
0749-0690/13/$ – see front matter © 2013 Elsevier Inc. All rights reserved.

of as too high risk. As a result, elderly candidates are now the fastest growing cohort of patients being waitlisted and transplanted. During the last 2 decades, waitlisings and transplants in candidates older than 65 years has increased by more than 5 fold.[2] The number of younger transplant recipients with functioning allografts reaching geriatric age has also increased. Thus, transplant physicians are caring for an ever growing geriatric kidney transplant population on chronic immunosuppression.

Aging is associated with functional and phenotypic changes in the immune system collectively referred to as immunosenescence. This process has effects on all the limbs of the immune system including cellular, humoral, and innate immunity. Although this aging process may have benefits with regard to transplantation by reducing the rate of organ rejection and promoting organ accommodation, the loss of effector function associated with immunosenescence places these patients at higher risk of serious infection and cancer, which is exacerbated by immunosuppression. Aging is also associated with changes in the pharmacokinetics and pharmacodynamics of drugs. Therefore, the elderly organ transplant recipient presents unique challenges with regard to immunosuppression.

Aging is also associated with functional decline in other organs systems and the accumulation of diseases that may affect outcomes after transplantation. Proper patient selection in the elderly is critical because surgery and the institution of immunosuppression have the potential to shorten life expectancy in candidates with higher levels of comorbidity. Elderly patients, who are prone to cognitive decline, may have more difficulty managing the complex medical regimens necessary for a successful kidney transplant. Cardiopulmonary diseases may increase both their perioperative and long-term mortality. Frailty and functional decline not only produce worse outcomes but also limit the quality of life benefits seen with kidney transplantation. In summary, elderly candidates present a more complex risk benefit equation with regard to kidney transplantation. Nonetheless, when properly selected and carefully transplanted, the elderly benefit from transplantation in many of the same ways as younger recipients.

AGING AND CELLULAR IMMUNITY

Understanding the functional changes to the immune system that occur with age is critical to the care of the elderly transplant recipient. This article is not an exhaustive review of the basic science of the aged immune system, and the author encourages readers who are interested in a more in-depth review of this topic to read the review articles cited in the paper. It has long been recognized that aging is associated with an increase in the risk of infection, reduced response to vaccination, and higher levels of autoantibody production.[3] More recently, the functional and phenotypic changes in the cellular immune system with aging have been better characterized. The hallmarks of aging in cellular immunity include thymic involution with a decline in the number of naïve T-cells, an increase in the number of memory cells associated with an increase in cytokine production, and a dysfunctional accumulation of activated effector cells of limited T-cell repertoire occupying the T-cell space.[3-8]

Thymopoiesis is critical for the health of the immune system through its generation of a broad repertoire of diverse T-cell receptors that can react with new potential antigens. Although thymopoiesis continues throughout life at some level, thymic involution associated with aging results in a decrease in the absolute numbers of naïve T-cells produced. This diminished export rate is insufficient to replace naïve T-cells lost daily in the periphery. The limited number of naïve T-cells leads to a gradual loss of repertoire diversity and hence potential impairment of immune response.

Associated with the decrease in absolute numbers of naïve T-cells is an increase in memory T-cells with defined cytokine phenotype and production. Two mechanisms appear to be responsible for the increase in the number of memory T-cells. The first is age-related accumulation of memory responses following antigen stimulation, and the second occurs as a result of homeostatic proliferation. Homeostatic proliferation is a process that replenishes the "fullness" of the T-cell compartment and occurs anytime a depletion of the peripheral compartment occurs due to either aging, viral infection, or depleting drugs such as induction agents in transplantation. Not only are the memory T-cells increased but repeated observations demonstrate elevated levels of pro-inflammatory cytokines (interferon-gamma, tumor necrosis factor-alpha) are produced by these memory cells contributing to the overall state of pro-inflammation seen in many elderly.

The final change associated with aging is the accumulation of activated effector cells of limited T-cell repertoire. Most of these cells are clonally expanded populations of cells reactive to a limited number of viruses, usually Cytomegalovirus and Epstein-Barr virus. These cells also have shortened telomeres and limited proliferative capacity and respond with only low levels of interferon-gamma when stimulated by viral antigens.

Another consequence of the aging cellular immune system with importance to transplantation is the reduced capacity for immune reconstitution after cytoreductive therapy. Lymphoreductive therapies such as polyclonal or monoclonal antilymphocyte globulins are agents commonly used in transplantation for induction. These agents lead to profound peripheral lymphopenia. With age, the recovery of normal lymphocyte levels after cytoreductive therapy is progressively retarded. Studies in bone marrow transplants have shown that the generation of naïve T-cells via thymopoiesis is inversely proportional to age, and the recovery of the naïve T-cell population is severely compromised after the fifth decade of life. Homeostatic proliferation of the remaining populations of cells leads to excess numbers of memory and terminally differentiated effector T-cells. This T-cell phenotype has the same characteristics of that seen with immunosenescence, suggesting that T-cell depleting therapies may cause "premature aging" of the cellular immune system.

AGING AND HUMORAL IMMUNITY

Similar to the changes in cellular immunity, with aging humoral immunity also appears to develop functional and phenotypic changes, which appear to impair humoral immune response.[9] Animal data suggest that B lymphopoiesis in the bone marrow decreases with age leading to a decreased output of new naïve B-cells to the periphery. Homeostatic proliferation of existing antigen-experienced B-cells both to environmental antigens and self-appear to fill the void in peripheral niches associated with the decline in naïve B-cells. It is thought that the shift in cellular constitution of peripheral lymphoid organs from naïve to antigen-experienced cells causes the decline in humoral immunity seen with aging and not functional defects in individual B-cells; individual B-cells retain their ability to produce antibody. The lack of sufficient populations of naïve b-cells and the reliance on existing antigen-experienced B-cells reduce the quality of antibody response because of a more limited repertoire of B-cell receptor clones. This hypothesis is supported by the fact that antibodies produced by a similar antigenic challenge had lower affinity and avidity in aged versus young animals.

The lower affinity humoral response seen in aged animals suggests that aging is associated with impairment of somatic hypermutation. This phenomenon occurs at the geminal centers, and there is evidence that the number and size of geminal centers declines with aging. T-cell help also appears to be impaired in aging animals contributing to the suboptimal humoral response. Taken together, the ability of the elderly to mount a humoral response to antigen stimulation is reduced.

AGING AND INNATE IMMUNITY

The innate immune system is comprised of a variety of immune cells important in primary immune defense including neutrophils, natural killer cells, monocytes, macrophages, and dendritic cells. These cells mediate the earliest interactions with pathogens and allograft tissue. Aging is associated with defects in activation of all these cell types that have been linked to compromised signal transduction pathways.[10] Some of the decline in innate immunity may be compensated by the proinflammatory milieu seen with aging. Therefore, immunosenescence of the innate immune system may better be termed dysregulation rather than age-associated decline.

Neutrophils are the primary immune defense against bacteria, yeast, and fungal infections. Interestingly, age is not associated with a reduction in the number of neutrophils, and a robust neutrophilia in response to infection remains intact. Neutrophils, however, do show compromised microbiocidal function and impaired chemotaxis with aging. Aged neutrophils show reduced phagocytosis, which is in part mediated by reduced expression of Fc-gamma receptor. The impaired chemotaxis may increase bystander tissue damage and slow resolution of inflammation.

Natural killer cells are important for host defense against viral infections and some cancers. Aging is associated with an increase in natural killer cell numbers but with a decrease in cytotoxicity and cytokine and chemokine release. Similar to the natural killer cells, monocytes also increase in number with age but display age-associated decrease in function and cytokine production. Finally, dendritic cells appear to decrease in function as a result of aging.

ELDERLY PATIENT SURVIVAL AFTER KIDNEY TRANSPLANTATION

Given the strong influence of age on patient survival, it is not surprising that elderly recipients faired worse then younger cohorts (**Table 1**). Graft survival in the elderly was also reduced when compared with younger recipients, and this difference in graft survival is driven primarily by higher rates of death with graft function. Nonetheless, 64.7% of recipients aged 65 years were still alive for 5 years and 58.7% of grafts were functioning indicating acceptable outcomes from kidney transplantation in this population.

Notwithstanding the quality-of-life benefit seen in elderly kidney transplant recipients,[11–13] the single most important advantage of kidney transplantation over conventional dialysis is the significant survival benefit that kidney transplant patients experience when compared with patients on the waiting list on dialysis. In the landmark study by Wolfe and colleagues,[14] deceased donor kidney transplant recipients had, on average, a doubling of life expectancy from 10 to 20 years when compared with patients remaining on dialysis on the waiting list. This benefit was seen in all races, all diagnoses of ESRD and both genders. In their analysis, recipients aged 60 to 74 years also showed a benefit in survival with an increase in lifespan of approximately 4 years. When this subgroup was further divided into 3 age groups 60 to 64 years, 65 to 69 years, and 70 to 74 years, the benefit did diminish significantly from 4.3 years to 2.8 years and finally to 1.0 year, respectively.

In a more recent study, Rao and colleagues[15] examined the outcomes of 5667 elderly patients older than 70 years waitlisted between the years 1990 and 2004. They found a 41% reduction in risk of death in patients transplanted versus patient remaining on the waiting list. Their analysis also showed that the recipients of

Table 1
Patient and graft survival by recipient age

	Recipient Age 35–49 y	Recipient Age 50–64 y	Recipient Age ≥65 y
		All Donor Types	
Patient Survival			
1 y	97.3%	94.6%	91.4%
3 y	93.3%	87.0%	79.8%
5 y	88.6%	78.4%	64.7%
Graft Survival			
1 y	92.6%	90.6%	87.9%
3 y	84.4%	80.5%	74.3%
5 y	74.8%	69.5%	58.9%

Note: Survival rates are reported as percentages.
Data from Organ procurement and transplantation network (OPTN) and scientific registry of transplant recipients (SRTR). OPTN/SRTR 2011 annual data report. Department of Health and Human Services, Health Resources and Services Administration, Healthcare Systems Bureau, Division of Transplantation. 2012. Available at: http://optn.transplant.hrsa.gov/latestData/rptData.asp. Accessed April 25, 2013.

expanded criteria donor kidneys had a 25% reduction in the risk of death vis a vis patients remaining on the waiting list. Although the long-term risk was lower, the relative risk of mortality in the first 45 days was increased with a relative risk of death of 2.26, and equal risk of death occurred at 125 days post-transplant for a deceased donor recipient. Although the absolute risk of death is higher in elderly kidney transplant recipients, the relative risk profile was similar to that seen in the analysis by Wolfe and colleagues for all deceased donor recipients. Because of this increase in early risk of death, the patient transplanted with a deceased donor did worse as a population until 1.8 years, at which time the survival curves crossed leading to the long-term survival advantage seen in the transplanted population (**Fig. 1**).

Although these studies reveal a survival advantage to kidney transplantation that extends into the eighth decade, it is important to remember that the elderly cohorts studied were highly selected. Recent data from the US Renal Data System show that less than 4% of prevalent ESRD patients older than 70 years are listed for

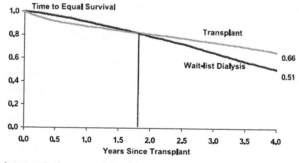

Fig. 1. Cumulative survival curves for elderly deceased donor transplant recipients and elderly wait-listed dialysis patients. (*From* Rao PS, Merion RM, Ashby VB, et al. Renal transplantation in elderly patients older than 70 years of age: results from the scientific registry of transplant recipients. Transplantation 2007;83(8):1069–74; with permission.)

transplant, indicating the highly selected nature of this group.[1] The difficult question that transplant professionals must grapple with is who is an appropriate elderly candidate for transplantation. This survival benefit may not extend to patients with serious comorbidities. Unfortunately, no good studies exist regarding outcomes based on comorbidity profiles.

ACUTE AND CHRONIC REJECTION

Most data suggests that the risk of acute rejection in the elderly is reduced. Two large registry analyses of US transplant data both showed a progressive decline in the rate of early acute rejection with age. In the first study, whereas the early rejection rate for 18-year-olds to 29-year-olds was 28%, recipients older than 65 years had a rejection rate of 19.7%.[16] Similarly, in a second study the rate of rejection for patients who are 18 years old was 28% compared to only 14% in recipients older than 70 years.[17]

In contrast, controversy exists with regard to the impact of age on chronic rejection. In an early study by Meier-Kriesche and colleagues,[18] elderly patient appeared to be at increased risk of chronic graft failure. In a later study, Keith and colleagues[19] showed that elderly patients were at lower risk for chronic graft loss after 6 months, suggesting that the elderly may be less prone to chronic rejection or chronic allograft nephropathy. Both these analyses were of US registry data with their inherent weakness with regard to accurate classification of graft loss. At least 4 single center studies support the latter observation that elderly kidney transplant recipients are less prone to this cause of graft loss, suggesting that loss of immune competence with age may reduce the incidence of chronic rejection.[20–23]

The most important cause of graft loss in the elderly population is death with graft function.[24,25] Most elderly candidates do not outlive the function of their grafts. Deceased donor kidneys have a broad spectrum of survival potential depending most importantly on age of the donor. Kidneys from younger donors last longer than those transplanted from older donors. Given the shortage of donor organs, in order to improve the utility of organ use, some have advocated for age matching the donor and recipient (ie, old donor to old recipient and young donor to young recipient).[26] This approach leads to an overall improvement in survival of the population transplanted, but modeling of this approach to organ allocation in the United States resulted in fewer elderly transplants given the age demographic of the donor population.[27] Also, a study looking at age matching and outcomes revealed that elderly candidates benefit with regard to patient survival if they receive a young donor kidney versus an older donor kidney, indicating that even patients with diminished survival potential benefit from a younger donor organ.[28]

ORGAN SELECTION IN THE ELDERLY TRANSPLANT CANDIDATE

Selection of an appropriate donor kidney for the elderly patient is complex. What is clear from the available research is that living donor kidney transplant provides the best outcomes for elderly transplant recipients. Living donor transplantation is associated with lower perioperative mortality and the best long-term outcomes among elderly transplant recipients (**Fig. 2**).[29] For patients in regions with long waiting times for deceased donor organs, this may be their only realistic opportunity for transplantation. In spite of the significant benefits of living donor transplantation, the elderly have the lowest rate of living donor transplantation among different age groups.[2] One of the largest impediments to living donor transplant in the elderly is their reluctance to accept organs from their children or other younger members of society. Also, some have questioned the utility of using potentially long lived grafts in

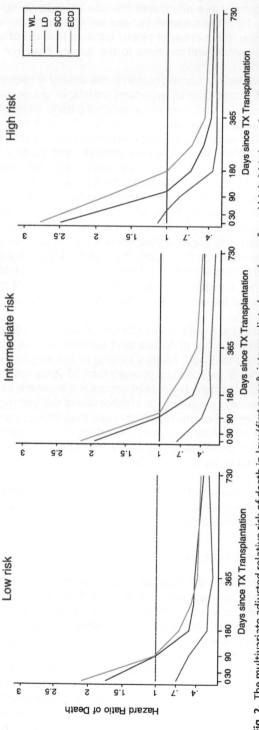

Fig. 2. The multivariate adjusted relative risk of death in low (*first panel*), intermediate (*second panel*), and high (*third panel*) cardiovascular risk elderly patients. In each panel, red is the living donor recipients, purple is the standard criteria deceased donor recipients, and the green is the expanded criteria deceased donor recipients. The blue line is the comparison to the risk of death on the waiting list. As can be seen, the type of donor affects the relative risk of early death, with living donors having the lowest risk of early death. Long-term risk was better for all types of donors over remaining on the waiting list. (*From* Gill JS, Schaeffner E, Chadban S, et al. Quantification of the early risk of death in elderly kidney transplant recipients. Am J Transplant 2013;13(2):427–32; with permission.)

recipients with diminished survival potential. In order to improve living donor transplantation in the elderly some have advocated the use of older living donors.[30] Indeed, older living donors have been shown to have acceptable outcomes for this population.[31–34] Unfortunately, the number of elderly patients who are of acceptable health for living donation is small, and the risks to the donors have not been well quantified.

The other major option for kidney transplantation in the elderly is deceased donor kidney transplant, either standard criteria, expanded criteria, or donor after cardiac death. As discussed earlier, both standard and expanded criteria donors have been shown to provide a survival advantage over continue dialysis, the former more than the latter. The decision to consider accepting an expanded criteria donor kidney is largely based on the local waiting time, age, race/ethnicity, and cause of renal failure.[35] For those candidates who reside in a donor service area with short waiting times, it may be preferable to wait for a standard criteria kidney with its better long-term outcomes. However, for most elderly candidates who live in donor service areas with longer waiting times and especially those with diabetes mellitus or other comorbid conditions associated with shortened survival on dialysis, accepting an expanded criteria donor has been shown to improve their chances of transplantation with its attendant benefits. Unfortunately, as the organ shortage for kidney transplantation worsens and waiting times increase, for many elderly there will be de facto exclusion from deceased donor kidney transplantation due to their poor survival potential on dialysis. Indeed, it is projected that more than 50% of elderly waitlisted patients will not be transplanted.[36]

No studies exist assessing the merits of transplanting elderly candidates with donors after cardiac death. The number of donors after cardiac death is increasing as a portion of the deceased donor pool.[2] Studies looking at the long-term outcomes of these kidneys indicate that at least donors younger than 50 years have similar outcomes to that seen in standard criteria brain dead donors in the general kidney transplant population.[37] These kidneys are subject to a higher rate of delayed graft function, which may affect the well being of elderly recipients more than their younger counterparts. Although standard criteria kidneys have a rate of delayed graft function (defined as dialysis in the first week post-transplant) of approximately 20%, donors after cardiac death have a rate that is double that of 40%.[37] Delayed graft function is associated with an increase in morbidity and mortality in the peri-operative period, and elderly recipients are more prone to these negative outcomes.[38] Whether this risk with donors after cardiac death deceases the survival benefit of kidney transplantation in this population has yet to be elucidated.

IMMUNOSUPPRESSION IN THE ELDERLY

It is generally accepted that the immune system loses competence with age as a consequence of immunosenescence. Currently the clinical tools for assessing immune competence are lacking, and no studies assessing immune phenotypes and outcome exist. Additionally, the elderly population is not monolithic but heterogeneous with respect to the competence of the immune system, and physiologic age rather than chronologic age may be a better predictor of immune function. As a population, however, it is clear that elderly transplant recipients are at significantly higher risk for cancers and fatal infections and appear to have lower rates of acute rejection, indicating that as a group they are less immunocompetent than younger recipients.[39,40] Unfortunately, there are no prospective studies comparing maintenance immunosuppressive protocols in the elderly, so little is known regarding the optimal maintenance immunosuppression in this population. Most transplant professionals believe that lower levels of maintenance immunosuppression are necessary in this population to maintain allograft accommodation when compared with younger recipients, but studies comparing dosing and immunosuppression composition are lacking.

Just as trials in maintenance immunosuppression are lacking in the elderly so are induction immunosuppression trials. There are 2 schools of thought with regard to induction in the elderly. The first is premised on the contention that immunocompetence and the risk of rejection wanes with age while the risk of infection and cancer increase. Minimizing the potency of or eliminating induction in the elderly recipient is advocated. The second school of thought believes that rejection is more poorly tolerated in the elderly, and they would advocate potent induction to prevent this complication. Indeed, older retrospective data support the contention that elderly patients tolerate rejection more poorly than younger recipients.[41] However, these data come from an era when rejection rates were much higher, maintenance immunosuppression was less potent, and prophylaxis against cytomegalovirus was poor. Finally, a retrospective study on induction therapy in the elderly supports both positions but for different immunologic risk patients.[42] This study stratified the risk of graft failure and rejection based on both donor and recipient factors. Although rejection rates were lower in all patients who received lymphocyte depleting agents when compared with those who received interleukin 2 receptor antagonists or no induction, only the candidates with high immunologic risk for rejection and who received high-risk donors saw an improved graft survival with lymphocyte depletion agents. For elderly candidates at low immunologic risk for rejection and low-risk donor organs, no benefit was seen with regard to graft and patient survival. Therefore, a more nuanced approach to induction with attention to pretransplant rejection risk and donor quality may be necessary to optimize outcomes in the elderly.

More is know about the pharmacokinetics of drugs in the elderly. In general, aging is associated with decreased rates of drug metabolism. This has been confirmed with studies of cyclosporine dosing that show elderly individuals require lower doses of cyclosporine to achieve the same serum trough levels as seen in younger recipients, indicating a diminishment of metabolism of the drug.[43] Pharmacokinetic studies of other commonly used immunosuppressives in the elderly are lacking, but many of the principles for dosing medication in the elderly are adopted with the use of immunosuppressive agents. Following the mantra of low and slow for dosing of immunosuppression is prudent in elderly transplant recipient because they are more prone to side effects and toxicity of medications. Also, comorbid conditions more commonly seen in elderly recipients, such as familial tremor, osteoporosis, diabetes mellitus, skin cancers, hypertension, or hyperlipidemia, can be exacerbated by immunosuppressive medications, and judicious choices and dosing of immunosuppressive medications may help ameliorate these conditions.

Unfortunately, little is known about longitudinal management of immunosuppression over the lifespan of the recipient. Improving graft outcomes in kidney transplantation means increasing numbers of transplant recipients surviving into their geriatric years, and the number of new geriatric recipients is growing every year. Studies of immunosenescence in the elderly would suggest that the immune system declines in function with age, but it is not known whether this should be accompanied by a reduction in immunosuppression or at which age the reduction should take place. For the most part, longitudinal management of immunosuppression is reactive rather than proactive, that is to say that changes in immunosuppression typically occur only after an immunosuppression complication has occurred such as a cancer or serious infection.

SELECTION OF THE ELDER TRANSPLANT CANDIDATE

Several factors must be considered when determining the candidacy of an elderly patient, including health status, cognitive function, frailty, adequacy of social support systems, finances, and local waiting time for deceased donor kidney transplant. Although there is no absolute age cut-off for consideration of kidney transplant, the overall health of the patient is an important consideration when selecting elderly candidates for kidney transplantation. Because elderly patients are more likely to have comorbid conditions that may affect their candidacy and outcome after transplant, a careful medical evaluation is imperative. Patients need to be carefully screened for cancer and chronic infections that may be affected by immunosuppression. Also, a thorough evaluation of the cardiovascular system is important to determine both a candidate's immediate risk of perioperative event and their overall long-term mortality risk. The elderly have the highest rates of death of any age group on the waiting list.[2] A substantial amount of resources are used to place and maintain patients on the waiting list; placing elderly candidates with many comorbid conditions may not be indicated and waste resources needed elsewhere. No hard and fast rules for determining candidacy for kidney transplant exist with regard to age, and transplant programs may list candidates at their own discretion depending on waiting times, comorbid conditions, and local listing criteria.

Cognitive function is an important factor that must be taken into consideration. Aging is associated with increasing incidence of cognitive impairment and Alzheimer disease. If there is suspicion of a cognitive deficit, neuropsychologic testing may be indicated in order to rule out early dementia that is generally a contraindication for transplantation.

Even subtle cognitive deficits may impair a candidate's ability to follow the complex medical regimens necessary for successful transplant. Therefore, a thorough investigation of cognitive function is an important part of any geriatric evaluation.

Frailty is being increasingly recognized as a risk factor for poor survival on dialysis and may also be a risk factor for poor outcomes after transplantation. Frailty appears to be associated with an increase in delay graft function after kidney transplantation and poor outcomes after elective surgery.[44,45] However, the utility of frailty in predicting transplant outcomes awaits further research.

Psychosocial factors are also important when considering elderly candidates for kidney transplantation. Elderly candidates may have inadequate social support due to death or illness of a spouse and lack of available family or friends for help. Transplantation is a complex endeavor that requires frequent visits to the doctor, complex medical regimens, and multiple medications for success. Patients with inadequate support systems are more prone to medical noncompliance, which can result in poor outcomes. For patients with inadequate social support, it may be preferable to maintain the patient on in-center hemodialysis where they have a built-in support system, which prevents the isolation that may accompany kidney transplantation.

Finances may be another impediment for elderly patients. Although in the United States patients older than 65 years generally qualify for Medicare, this only covers 80% of the cost of transplantation. Unless they have supplement insurance to cover the 20% not covered by Medicare, patients may be unable to afford the cost of the surgery and medications. A careful financial screening is an important component of the screening process for kidney transplantation in the elderly.

Finally, for candidates without living donors, local waiting times are an important consideration for candidacy. The current organ allocation system in the United States is divided geographically into 58 donor services areas. For the most part, organs procured within a donor service area are also allocated locally to candidates listed in that donor service area. This system has led to large geographic variations in waiting times for deceased donor kidneys.[46] Although the shortest waiting time areas have median waiting times of a little more than a year, those from the longest waiting time areas are as high as 8 years. Within the donor service areas, waiting time also varies by blood type, with O and B blood types having the longest waiting times and A and AB the shortest. Because older candidates in general have a shorter survival time on dialysis than younger candidates and as a result a smaller window of opportunity for transplantation, opportunities to transplant the elderly are greater in shorter waiting time donor service areas and in candidates with favorable blood types. Listing an elderly candidate without a living donor, in a long waiting time donor service area, and with an unfavorable blood type, who has little chance of surviving to transplantation, may not be indicated.

SUMMARY

Whereas kidney transplantation is the treatment of choice for most young candidates due to its large survival advantage over dialysis, the risk benefit equation with regard to kidney transplantation is more complex in the geriatric candidate. Aging is associated with functional changes in the immune system and the accumulation of morbidity that affect the outcomes of kidney transplantation. For elderly candidates who are frail and have high levels of comorbidity, kidney transplantation may shorten life expectancy over continued dialysis. To date, however, among the highly selected population of geriatric kidney transplant recipients, both a quality of life and survival benefit over dialysis have been demonstrated. Therefore, properly selected geriatric candidates benefit from transplantation in many of the same ways as younger candidates. Unfortunately, due to increasing demand for kidneys and ever increasing waiting times, deceased donor kidney transplant as an option for the elderly is becoming more difficult due to their limited survival on dialysis. The organ shortage raises difficult questions regarding allocation of a scarce resource and how patients are selected for listing. There is no age limit for consideration of kidney transplantation, and the selection process remains largely subjective and at the whim of the transplant program. Given the growing geriatric ESRD population, not only is better research necessary to define those geriatric subgroups that benefit most from kidney transplantation but also is public discourse on how we allocate this scarce resource in an aging population.

REFERENCES

1. U S renal data system, USRDS 2012 annual data report: Atlas of chronic kidney disease and end-stage renal disease in the United States, national institutes of health, national institute of diabetes and digestive and kidney diseases, Bethesda, MD, 2012. Bethesda (MD): National Institutes of Health, National Institute of Diabetes and Digestive and Kidney Diseases; 2012.
2. Organ procurement and transplantation network (OPTN) and scientific registry of transplant recipients (SRTR). OPTN/SRTR 2011 annual data report. Department of Health and Human Services, Health Resources and Services Administration, Healthcare Systems Bureau, Division of Transplantation. 2012. Available at: http://optn.transplant.hrsa.gov/latestData/rptData.asp. Accessed April 25, 2013.
3. Weiskopf D, Weinberger B, Grubeck-Loebenstein B. The aging of the immune system. Transpl Int 2009;22(11):1041–50.

4. Flores KG, Li J, Sempowski GD, et al. Analysis of the human thymic perivascular space during aging. J Clin Invest 1999;104(8):1031–9.
5. George AJ, Ritter MA. Thymic involution with ageing: obsolescence or good housekeeping? Immunol Today 1996;17(6):267–72.
6. Fagnoni FF, Vescovini R, Passeri G, et al. Shortage of circulating naive CD8(+) T cells provides new insights on immunodeficiency in aging. Blood 2000;95(9): 2860–8.
7. Effros RB, Cai Z, Linton PJ. CD8 T cells and aging. Crit Rev Immunol 2003; 23(1–2):45–64.
8. Pfister G, Weiskopf D, Lazuardi L, et al. Naive T cells in the elderly: are they still there? Ann N Y Acad Sci 2006;1067:152–7.
9. Johnson SA, Cambier JC. Ageing, autoimmunity and arthritis: senescence of the B cell compartment - implications for humoral immunity. Arthritis Res Ther 2004; 6(4):131–9.
10. Shaw AC, Joshi S, Greenwood H, et al. Aging of the innate immune system. Curr Opin Immunol 2010;22(4):507–13.
11. Humar A, Denny R, Matas AJ, et al. Graft and quality of life outcomes in older recipients of a kidney transplant. Exp Clin Transplant 2003;1(2):69–72.
12. Cornella C, Brustia M, Lazzarich E, et al. Quality of life in renal transplant patients over 60 years of age. Transplant Proc 2008;40(6):1865–6.
13. Laupacis A, Keown P, Pus N, et al. A study of the quality of life and cost-utility of renal transplantation. Kidney Int 1996;50(1):235–42.
14. Wolfe RA, Ashby VB, Milford EL, et al. Comparison of mortality in all patients on dialysis, patients on dialysis awaiting transplantation, and recipients of a first cadaveric transplant. N Engl J Med 1999;341(23):1725–30.
15. Rao PS, Merion RM, Ashby VB, et al. Renal transplantation in elderly patients older than 70 years of age: results from the scientific registry of transplant recipients. Transplantation 2007;83(8):1069–74.
16. Meier-Kriesche HU, Ojo A, Hanson J, et al. Increased immunosuppressive vulnerability in elderly renal transplant recipients. Transplantation 2000;69(5):885–9.
17. Tullius SG, Milford E. Kidney allocation and the aging immune response. N Engl J Med 2011;364(14):1369–70.
18. Meier-Kriesche H, Ojo AO, Arndorfer JA, et al. Recipient age as an independent risk factor for chronic renal allograft failure. Transplant Proc 2001;33(1–2):1113–4.
19. Keith DS, Cantarovich M, Paraskevas S, et al. Recipient age and risk of chronic allograft nephropathy in primary deceased donor kidney transplant. Transpl Int 2006;19(8):649–56.
20. Pirsch JD, Ploeg RJ, Gange S, et al. Determinants of graft survival after renal transplantation. Transplantation 1996;61(11):1581–6.
21. Stoves J, Newstead CG. Variability of cyclosporine exposure and its relevance to chronic allograft nephropathy: a case-control study. Transplantation 2002;74(12): 1794–7.
22. Sijpkens YW, Doxiadis II, van Kemenade FJ, et al. Chronic rejection with or without transplant vasculopathy. Clin Transplant 2003;17(3):163–70.
23. Lietz K, Lewandowski Z, Lao M, et al. Pretransplant and early posttransplant predictors of chronic allograft nephropathy in cadaveric kidney allograft–a single-center analysis of 1112 cases. Transpl Int 2004;17(2):78–88.
24. Oniscu GC, Brown H, Forsythe JL. How old is old for transplantation? Am J Transplant 2004;4(12):2067–74.
25. Qiu J, Cai J, Terasaki PL. Death with a functioning graft in kidney transplant recipients. Clin Transpl 2004;379–86.

26. de Fijter JW. Counselling the elderly between hope and reality. Nephrol Dial Transplant 2011;26(7):2079–81.
27. Singh N, Nori U, Pesavento T. Kidney transplantation in the elderly. Curr Opin Organ Transplant 2009;14(4):380–5.
28. Keith DS, Demattos A, Golconda M, et al. Effect of donor recipient age match on survival after first deceased donor renal transplantation. J Am Soc Nephrol 2004; 15(4):1086–91.
29. Gill JS, Schaeffner E, Chadban S, et al. Quantification of the early risk of death in elderly kidney transplant recipients. Am J Transplant 2013;13(2):427–32.
30. Gill JS, Gill J, Rose C, et al. The older living kidney donor: part of the solution to the organ shortage. Transplantation 2006;82(12):1662–6.
31. Young A, Kim SJ, Speechley MR, et al. Accepting kidneys from older living donors: impact on transplant recipient outcomes. Am J Transplant 2011;11(4): 743–50.
32. Nanovic L, Kaplan B. The advantage of live-donor kidney transplantation in older recipients. Nat Clin Pract Nephrol 2009;5(1):18–9.
33. Lim WH, Clayton P, Wong G, et al. Outcomes of kidney transplantation from older living donors. Transplantation 2013;95(1):106–13.
34. Gill J, Bunnapradist S, Danovitch GM, et al. Outcomes of kidney transplantation from older living donors to older recipients. Am J Kidney Dis 2008;52(3):541–52.
35. Merion RM, Ashby VB, Wolfe RA, et al. Deceased-donor characteristics and the survival benefit of kidney transplantation. JAMA 2005;294(21):2726–33.
36. Schold J, Srinivas TR, Sehgal AR, et al. Half of kidney transplant candidates who are older than 60 years now placed on the waiting list will die before receiving a deceased-donor transplant. Clin J Am Soc Nephrol 2009;4(7):1239–45.
37. Locke JE, Segev DL, Warren DS, et al. Outcomes of kidneys from donors after cardiac death: implications for allocation and preservation. Am J Transplant 2007;7(7):1797–807.
38. Gill JS, Pereira BJ. Death in the first year after kidney transplantation: implications for patients on the transplant waiting list. Transplantation 2003;75(1):113–7.
39. Meier-Kriesche HU, Ojo AO, Hanson JA, et al. Exponentially increased risk of infectious death in older renal transplant recipients. Kidney Int 2001;59(4):1539–43.
40. Engels EA, Pfeiffer RM, Fraumeni JF Jr, et al. Spectrum of cancer risk among US solid organ transplant recipients. JAMA 2011;306(17):1891–901.
41. Meier-Kriesche HU, Srinivas TR, Kaplan B. Interaction between acute rejection and recipient age on long-term renal allograft survival. Transplant Proc 2001; 33(7–8):3425–6.
42. Gill J, Sampaio M, Gill JS, et al. Induction immunosuppressive therapy in the elderly kidney transplant recipient in the United States. Clin J Am Soc Nephrol 2011;6(5):1168–78.
43. Jacobson PA, Schladt D, Oetting WS, et al. Lower calcineurin inhibitor doses in older compared to younger kidney transplant recipients yield similar troughs. Am J Transplant 2012;12(12):3326–36.
44. Garonzik-Wang JM, Govindan P, Grinnan JW, et al. Frailty and delayed graft function in kidney transplant recipients. Arch Surg 2012;147(2):190–3.
45. Makary MA, Segev DL, Pronovost PJ, et al. Frailty as a predictor of surgical outcomes in older patients. J Am Coll Surg 2010;210(6):901–8.
46. Ashby VB, Kalbfleisch JD, Wolfe RA, et al. Geographic variability in access to primary kidney transplantation in the united states, 1996-2005. Am J Transplant 2007;7(5 Pt 2):1412–23.

Slowing the Aging Process

Jocelyn Wiggins, B.M., B.Ch, MRCP[a],*, Markus Bitzer, MD[b]

KEYWORDS

- Aging • Chronic kidney disease • Genetic pathways • Cellular processes

KEY POINTS

- Aging is a complex biological process controlled by genetic pathways.
- Cellular pathways are modified during aging resulting in phenotype instability and loss of specialization.
- Cellular organelles also exhibit signs of aging and inefficiency.
- Calorie restriction is currently the only proven intervention to slow or reverse the pathologies that develop with aging, although the new knowledge shows hope for interventions for the future.

INTRODUCTION

Slowing the aging process has been a dream since the dawn of civilization. Tales of the fountain of youth have appeared in recorded writings and artwork in every culture and civilization for which historical data are available. Research into the aging process, however, is very new. For many years this research was believed to be futile, because aging was thought to be the natural and inevitable consequence of a life of wear and tear. The idea that aging could be influenced by the genetic code and had a modifiable biologic component is less than 20 years old. During this time, aging has come to be understood as a complex biologic process controlled by signaling pathways and transcription factors. Similar attitudes pervade the field of nephrology. Much vigorous debate exists within the renal community about whether a decline in renal function with age represents normal aging or kidney disease.[1,2]

GENETIC PATHWAYS OF AGING

Research into the biologic basis of aging was sparked by a chance finding in 1993 by Cynthia Kenyon and colleagues.[3] While studying the biology of the nematode *Caenorhabditis elegans*, she discovered a spontaneous gene mutation that prolonged the worm's life by one-third. This first gene was called daf-2 and mutations resulted in worms that were healthy, active, and fertile but lived much longer than the wild-type controls. In 1997, a different group cloned daf-2 and showed it to be the insulin

[a] Division of Geriatrics, Internal Medicine, University of Michigan, Ann Arbor, MI 48109, USA;
[b] Division of Nephrology, Internal Medicine, University of Michigan, Ann Arbor, MI 48109, USA
* Corresponding author.
E-mail address: wiggi@umich.edu

Clin Geriatr Med 29 (2013) 721–730
http://dx.doi.org/10.1016/j.cger.2013.05.009
0749-0690/13/$ – see front matter © 2013 Elsevier Inc. All rights reserved.

receptor family member insulin-like growth factor 1 (IGF-1).[4] Mutations in other insulin pathway family members have since been shown to have similar effects on longevity. Inhibiting IGF pathways extends lifespan through changes in gene expression in multiple other pathways, and these are reviewed in detail elsewhere.[5] Similar lifespan extension was soon shown for mutations in other genes within the same signaling pathway. This pathway affects expression of a DNA FOXO transcription factor that controls expression of activity in multiple metabolic pathways, which ultimately results in lifespan extension. The initial thought was that a process that worked in a small simple organism, such as C elegans, was unlikely to have a parallel in highly complex larger organisms. However, manipulation of this pathway has now been successfully used to extend lifespan in multiple organisms, including mice.[6] Although experimentally modulating activity in this pathway is clearly not possible in humans, mutations affecting activity in IGF-1 signaling have been shown in cohorts of centenarians.[7] This pathway has also been shown to play a role in the longevity response to calorie restriction.

In the 20 years since this seminal discovery, 3 other gene pathways have been added to the list of agents capable of modifying the aging process, including TOR signaling (target of rapamycin). TOR inhibition increases lifespan in all experimental models, from yeast to mammals.[5] It is the pathway that is implicated in calorie restriction, and if a TOR transgenic animal is calorie-restricted, further extension of lifespan does not occur.[8,9] This pathway interacts with pathways that control mRNA translation, autophagy, and mitochondrial metabolism. The exact mechanism whereby aging is slowed is still being elucidated, and currently no data exist on whether this pathway is implicated in aging in the kidney. As noted later, experiments are currently underway in mice to extend lifespan using rapamycin.[10] Clearly, careful thought will need to be given to the use of rapamycin for aging in humans in view of its many side effects. However, the significant work on this pathway holds promise for finding ways to slow age-related pathologies and facilitate healthy, disease-free aging.

The sirtuin pathways are believed to be the target of resveratrol, the much-touted "healthy ingredient" in red wine. Sirtuins are a broadly conserved family of enzymes found in all phyla of life, from the simplest to the most complex. These ancient proteins have a common biochemistry, which allows them to interact with NAD^+ (nicotinamide adenine dinucleotide) and deacetylated proteins. The first link with aging was the discovery of SIR2 (silent information regulator) in yeast, which controlled the healthy extension of lifespan.[11,12] Seven mammalian homologs exist: SIRT1 through SIRT7.[13] Knockouts of at least one family member, SIRT6, cause premature aging.[14] As this field continues to grow, new roles for these ubiquitous molecules are continually being added. They have been shown to be important in adaptation to low-nutrient conditions, mitochondrial function, DNA repair, neuronal survival, and the maintenance of a youthful pattern of gene survival. Which of these functions is responsible for the increase in lifespan is not yet clear. SIRT1, SIRT3, and SIRT6 are all induced by calorie restriction, suggesting a mechanism for the benefits seen in calorie-restricted animals. Research also implicates the sirtuins in metabolic dysfunction such as diabetes; cancer suppression; and cardiovascular disease, which is the world's leading cause of death.[14] This field is rapidly expanding field, but with no link to the kidney to date.

Klotho is a gene that characterizes an accelerated aging phenotype, named after the Greek goddess who spun the thread of life. The role of klotho in aging was an accidental finding published in 1997.[15] A group making a transgenic mouse had fortuitously inserted their transgene randomly into the promoter region of the klotho gene and produced a prematurely aged mouse that lived only 5% to 6% of the normal captive mouse lifespan. Subsequent work with an overexpressing model produced a mouse that lived 20% to 30% longer than the wild-type littermates.[16] *Klotho* is expressed as both a membrane protein and a secreted protein, primarily in the distal tubular cells of the kidney. Its primary role seems to be as a cofactor or coreceptor regulating fibroblast growth factor 23 signaling and activation of the ion channel TRPV5. It plays an important role in phosphorus homeostasis. Klotho promotes phosphate excretion, and its reduced expression is associated with ectopic calcification, increased concentrations of $1,25\ (OH)_2D_3$, hyperphosphatemia, and therapy-resistant hyperparathyroidism.[17,18] Although these functions are important in the context of renal disease, the aging phenotype seems to be modulated through the IGF-1 signaling pathway. Secreted klotho inhibits insulin/IGF-1 signaling, and klotho-deficient mice are hypoglycemic and highly insulin-sensitive. The klotho-overexpressing mice are IGF-1–resistant. This interaction with an evolutionary-conserved mechanism for regulating aging seems to confer the aging phenotype. Reduced expression of klotho has been observed in patients with chronic kidney disease. Some single nucleotide polymorphisms in human klotho are associated with altered lifespan and increased vascular disease.[19] Klotho is clearly an interesting protein with a role in the complications of chronic kidney disease, and maybe in the altered lifespan associated with this disease.

Currently, mTOR is the only gene specifically targeted as a novel way to retard aging. Laboratories are actively pursuing the IGF-1 and sirtuin pathways as potential targets. Mouse experiments are currently ongoing and attempting to slow the aging process using rapamycin (sirolimus) to interfere with *mTOR* signaling.[10] Results from this study so far are modest, with an increase in maximum lifespan of 14% for female mice and 9% for male mice. Although these results show promise for pharmacologic interventions to prevent age-related diseases, whether age-associated glomerulosclerosis can be slowed remains to be shown. The significant side-effect profile associated with rapamycin must also be considered.

DNA Damage and Progerias

Maintaining the integrity of DNA is essential for healthy cellular well-being. Mutations in DNA are the cause of many cancers and many accelerated aging processes. Mutations that lead to accelerated aging are usually localized to the genes responsible for DNA repair, replication, and transcription. The best studied of these premature aging syndromes, known as *progerias*, are caused by mutations in helicases, which are responsible for reading, checking, and repairing the integrity of DNA. Loss of function in helicases can result in defective replication, inefficient transcription, deficient mismatch repair, and chromosome rearrangements. Although none of the progeroid syndromes exactly matches physiologic aging, studies of these syndromes are yielding clues as to how DNA damage, which accumulates with age, may play a role in the aging process.[20] One report exists of kidney pathology related to progeria. It describes renal histopathology from 2 subjects who died of progeria. The younger subject, who died at aged 11 years, had no glomerulosclerosis, where the kidney from the 20-year-old subject showed focal renal scarring with focal glomerulosclerosis and associated tubular atrophy, similar to that seen in physiologic aging.[21] Studies of these genetic pathways and the cellular response to DNA instability have shown that the cell can switch on an antiaging response by suppressing metabolism and cell growth through the TOR pathway. Targeting DNA repair systems clearly represents a major biologic challenge, and is unlikely to result in novel therapeutics in the near future.

Telomeres

Telomeres are specialized structures at the ends of chromosomes. They are vital for chromosome stability and maintenance of chromosome length during cell division. Telomere length dictates cell lifespan, because each round of DNA replication results in successive telomere shortening, until the telomeres become critically shortened, resulting in cellular crisis. At least 2 barriers seem to exist that may alter replicative senescence for diploid cell types; one is premature telomere shortening and the other is an accumulation of environmental stress-imposed DNA damage, limiting the number of cell divisions to 10 to 15 instead of 50 or more in vitro. An excellent review by Campisi[22] outlines the current understanding of the relationship among cellular senescence, tumor suppression, and organism aging. How is this complex cell biology relevant to the kidney? Westhoff and colleagues[23] studied the role of telomeres in ischemia-reperfusion injury in telomerase-deficient mice. They compared fourth-generation mice with first- and second-generation mice. As the telomeres shortened through the generations, mice showed reduced proliferative capacity in tubular, glomerular, and interstitial cells. They were more vulnerable to acute kidney injury and less likely to regenerate tubular epithelium. They mimicked older patients, who are significantly more susceptible to acute renal injury and less likely to recover renal function after such an injury. Feest and colleagues[24] showed that a progressive age-dependent increase in acute kidney injury occurs after 60 years of age. Mortality also increases with age, and older patients who require dialysis have a mortality rate greater than 80%.[25] Rates of renal function recovery are 28% lower in patients older than 65 years.[26]

Understanding of the individual genes and pathways that can affect aging and age-associated declines in organ function is instructive. Altering gene function through genetic engineering, however, is currently beyond the scope of current medicine. Finding small molecule inhibitors or mimics to manipulate pathways are likely to be more productive at the current time. Many of the burdens of aging are related to chronic disease burden. Many of these diseases are driven by the transcription factor, nuclear factor kappa-B (NF-kB), including age-associated glomerulosclerosis.[27] Learning how to manipulate these drivers of aging-related disease without affecting the normal functions of organs is one of the major challenges of aging biology.

CELLULAR PROCESSES THAT CHANGE WITH AGE
Epigenetics

Every cell in the body has the same compliment of DNA. During nephrogenesis, regulatory genes partition the genome into active and inactive domains, a process called *epigenetics*. This process allows the specification and maintenance of cellular phenotype. The body has 2 basic cell types: stem cells that are undifferentiated and capable of self-renewal and pluripotency, and somatic cells, which comprise the distinctive individual cell types of each organ. As cell lineage and patterning occur under the control of regulatory genes, chromatin domains are defined through methylation and acetylation of histones. These domains may be activated or silenced to direct the cell fate. These changes initiate differentiation and are maintained from one cell generation to the next during cell division. Through the process of methylation and acetylation, these changes in the genome become both stable and heritable. In this way, cell lineage becomes established and phenotype is maintained. How does epigenetics affect aging in the kidney? In cells that turnover on a regular basis, these epigenetic mechanisms are renewed at each cell division. Podocytes probably do not replicate, and therefore they need to maintain their epigenetic characteristics throughout a lifetime. If their epigenetic marks are unstable over time, one would expect to see the loss of characteristic phenotypic proteins and/or expression of proteins that should have been silenced. In rat models of the aging glomerulus both of these processes are seen.[27] Using a genetic screening process in aging Fischer 344 rats, 92 glomerular genes were found that seemed to be silenced at 2 months but had robust expression by 24 months. The most striking example was prepronociceptin, a neurologic gene that has been characterized as a modulator in pain signaling pathways. It showed a greater than 80-fold increase in expression in the glomerulus between young and old rats, suggesting that this area of chromatin had been silenced during differentiation but had achieved expression because of failure of the epigenetic regulation with age. In contrast, nephrin, a podocyte-specific protein, showed a decline in expression in the same animals, again suggesting inefficiencies in epigenetic patterning with age. Epigenetic mechanisms are an attractive target for manipulation. Changing genes requires complicated genetic engineering. To master the control of epigenetics, one would be able to turn signaling pathways on or off and influence the outcomes of health and disease.

MicroRNAs

MicroRNAs (miRNAs) are one of the newest areas of research in regulatory biology. The first miRNA was discovered in 1993. They are single-stranded noncoding (nontranslated) RNA molecules of 22 to 25 nucleotides. They are expressed in the nucleus as a 70-base-pair stem-loop structure, which is cleaved into a short active form in the cytoplasm. Maintaining cellular and organismal homeostasis in an ever-changing and challenging environment requires the coordinated action of complex signaling pathways that balance the activity of damage and repair mechanisms in response to external and internal stressors. Discoveries in C elegans and mice have shown that miRNAs regulate key mechanisms of the stress response and aging process, including insulin/IGF, mTOR, and SIRT signaling, through functioning as feed-forward loops.[28,29] They act to repress mRNA and prevent translation. They have been shown to be extremely important in renal development, the regulation of gene expression in the kidney, and in renal diseases.[30] Harvey and colleagues[31] showed that disruption of miRNA leads to rapid end-stage kidney disease. miR-192 has been shown to play an important role in diabetic nephropathy. The role of miRNAs in cell senescence and aging is reviewed in detail by Grillari and colleagues.[32] Limited data currently exist on their role in aging in the kidney, but this role will be defined as more evidence accumulates about their role in differentiation, cellular function, and disease. Even though the mechanisms of miRNA:mRNA interactions are highly complex, far beyond the simple binding of an miRNA to a target mRNA, miRNAs may be attractive candidates to modulate the stress response and other tightly regulated signals because of their chemical structure, which may potentially allow inhibition and also repletion of miRNAs.

Organelles

Multiple intracellular organelles are believed to play a role in cell senescence and aging. Scientific evidence in the kidney supports a role for mitochondria and energy generation[33,34]; autophagy and the removal of damaged proteins[35,36]; and telomeres and cell replication.[22–26] A well-developed body of literature exists on the role of oxidants in the aging process.[37–39] Advanced glycation end products (AGEs) form when sugars are attached to the amino groups of proteins and nucleic acids. They are highly reactive and generate reactive oxygen species. AGEs can be derived from cellular oxidative metabolism and are increased in conditions such as diabetes, or they can be acquired through the diet.[40,41] High levels of oxidant stress are associated with all forms of age-related chronic disease, such as cardiovascular disease, cerebrovascular disease, chronic kidney disease, and diabetes.[42] They are also associated with increased markers of inflammation, such as fibrosis and macrophage infiltration. Elevated levels of oxidant stress and inflammation are associated with chronic kidney disease.[39] In addition to AGEs, oxidized lipids and lipoproteins also play a role in aging and kidney disease. Animal models of hypercholesterolemia, high-fat diets, and scavenger receptor defects are all associated with chronic kidney disease, atherosclerosis, and cardiovascular disease.[43,44] Studies of glomerular aging have shown significant changes in the expression of ceruloplasmin by parietal epithelial cells lining the Bowman capsule.[45] Ceruloplasmin is an antioxidant, and its expression increases 5-fold in ad lib–fed rats as they age. In calorie-restricted rats, ceruloplasmin protein expression increases less than 2-fold with age. Both the cell-associated alternately spliced variant and secreted variants of ceruloplasmin were expressed and can be detected in urine. Ceruloplasmin was therefore expressed by epithelial cells lining the Bowman capsule in direct proportion to known levels of oxidant activity (older age and high-calorie diet), and was secreted into the urine. This finding may well represent a protective mechanism within the kidney to reduce oxidant damage of the tubule by filtered oxidant load. Reducing oxidative damage can be approached through dietary modification and pharmacologic strategies. Several inhibitors of AGE formation exist, including aminoguanidine. Although animal models seemed encouraging, human trials have not shown any ability to prevent chronic kidney disease progression.[46,47] AGE cleaving agents, such as alagebrium, have shown promise in animals and humans.[48–52] Scientists have also been working on agents to block the AGE tissue receptor. Trials in humans are ongoing for a small molecule inhibitor of the AGE interaction with the receptor. Plant-derived polyphenolic compounds are also being studied for their antiglycative and antioxidant activity.

Calorie Restriction

Calorie restriction has been known to increase lifespan since 1935, when McCay and colleagues[53] published a rodent study showing that reducing calories without malnutrition extended both average and maximum life expectancy. Over the intervening years, work on calorie restriction and its mechanism was limited mainly to short-lived organisms, such as yeast, worms, and flies. In the 1980s, the National Institute on Aging (NIA) set up a series of studies in rodents to examine mechanisms of aging and the retardation of aging-associated pathologies, and not just extension of lifespan. The NIA developed specific colonies of aging mammals and systematically characterized the aging process in rodents, comparing ad lib–fed animals with their calorie-restricted littermates. They established guidelines for the nutritional management of calorie restriction, and continue to supply calorie-restricted animals and appropriate chow to funded projects.[54–56] Nadon[57] showed that calorie restriction could prevent, or at least delay, the onset of age-associated nephropathy. Most recently, Colman and colleagues[58] published the results of a 20-year longitudinal study of calorie restriction in primates. They observed the effect of calorie restriction on the resistance to age-associated illness and on mortality. They reported a 3-fold increase in the onset of age-associated diseases in ad lib–fed animals compared with calorie-restricted animals at any given age, and a significant increase in lifespan. They specifically studied the onset of diabetes, cancer, cardiovascular disease, and brain atrophy, because these are common diseases of aging in humans. Studies in rats have shown that calorie restriction reduces mesangial matrix expansion and proteinuria, and prevents the development of age-associated glomerulosclerosis.[59]

The effects of calorie restriction in humans is thoroughly reviewed by Redman and Ravussin.[60] Although these results are encouraging, calorie restriction itself is unlikely to be a realistic therapeutic option in humans.

The biology of human aging is a young but active and rapidly evolving field. Much progress has been made in elucidating the drivers of aging and aging-related pathologies, such as chronic kidney disease. Currently, there are as many questions as there are answers. The US Food and Drug Administration does not currently recognize aging as a disease. Therefore, until this changes, drugs will only be approved to treat age-associated diseases, and not the aging process itself. Once interventions are developed and shown to be safe and effective, this may change. Much work still needs to be done toward understanding the biologic process of aging. Interventions will lag far behind, as that knowledge is slowly translated into action.

REFERENCES

1. Glassock RJ, Oreopoulos DG. Aging and chronic kidney disease. Nephron Clin Pract 2011;119(Suppl 1):c1.
2. Winearls CG, Glassock RJ. Classification of chronic kidney disease in the elderly: pitfalls and errors. Nephron Clin Pract 2011;119(Suppl 1):c2–4.
3. Kenyon C, Chang J, Gensch E, et al. A C. elegans mutant that lives twice as long as wild type. Nature 1993;366(6454):461–4.
4. Kimura KD, Tissenbaum HA, Liu Y, et al. daf-2, an insulin receptor-like gene that regulates longevity and diapause in Caenorhabditis elegans. Science 1997; 277(5328):942–6.
5. Kenyon CJ. The genetics of ageing. Nature 2010;464(7288):504–12.
6. Yuan R, Tsaih SW, Petkova SB, et al. Aging in inbred strains of mice: study design and interim report on median lifespans and circulating IGF1 levels. Aging Cell 2009;8(3):277–87.
7. Pawlikowska L, Hu D, Huntsman S, et al. Association of common genetic variation in the insulin/IGF1 signaling pathway with human longevity. Aging Cell 2009; 8(4):460–72.
8. Kapahi P, Zid B. TOR pathway: linking nutrient sensing to life span. Sci Aging Knowledge Environ 2004;2004(36):PE34.
9. Kapahi P, Chen D, Rogers AN, et al. With TOR, less is more: a key role for the conserved nutrient-sensing TOR pathway in aging. Cell Metab 2010;11(6):453–65.
10. Harrison DE, Strong R, Sharp ZD, et al. Rapamycin fed late in life extends lifespan in genetically heterogeneous mice. Nature 2009;460(7253):392–5.
11. Sinclair DA, Guarente L. Extrachromosomal rDNA circles—a cause of aging in yeast. Cell 1997;91(7):1033–42.
12. Kaeberlein M, McVey M, Guarente L. The SIR2/3/4 complex and SIR2 alone promote longevity in Saccharomyces cerevisiae by two different mechanisms. Genes Dev 1999;13(19):2570–80.
13. Haigis MC, Sinclair DA. Mammalian sirtuins: biological insights and disease relevance. Annu Rev Pathol 2010;5:253–95.
14. Mostoslavsky R, Chua KF, Lombard DB, et al. Genomic instability and aging-like phenotype in the absence of mammalian SIRT6. Cell 2006; 124(2):315–29.
15. Kuro-o M, Matsumura Y, Aizawa H, et al. Mutation of the mouse klotho gene leads to a syndrome resembling ageing. Nature 1997;390:45–51.
16. Kurosu H, Yamamoto M, Clark JD, et al. Suppression of aging in mice by the hormone klotho. Science 2005;309:1829–33.

17. Wang Y, Sun Z. Current understanding of klotho. Ageing Res Rev 2009;8:43–51.
18. Kuro-o M. Klotho and aging. Biochim Biophys Acta 2009;1790:1049–58.
19. Arking DE, Krebsova A, Macek M Sr, et al. Association of human aging with a functional variant of klotho. Proc Natl Acad Sci U S A 2002;99:856–61.
20. Hoeijmakers JH. DNA damage, aging, and cancer. N Engl J Med 2009;361(15): 1475–85.
21. Delahunt B, Stehbens WE, Gilbert-Barness E, et al. Progeria kidney has abnormal mesangial collagen distribution. Pediatr Nephrol 2000;15(3–4):279–85.
22. Campisi J. Senescent cells, tumor suppression, and organismal aging: good citizens, bad neighbors. Cell 2005;120(4):513–22.
23. Westhoff JH, Schildhorn C, Jacobi C, et al. Telomere shortening reduces regenerative capacity after acute kidney injury. J Am Soc Nephrol 2010;21(2):327–36.
24. Feest TG, Round A, Hamad S. Incidence of severe acute renal failure in adults: results of a community based study. BMJ 1993;306(6876):481–3.
25. Wardle EN. Acute renal failure and multiorgan failure. Nephrol Dial Transplant 1994;9(Suppl 4):104–7.
26. Schmitt R, Coca S, Kanbay M, et al. Recovery of kidney function after acute kidney injury in the elderly: a systematic review and meta-analysis. Am J Kidney Dis 2008;52(2):262–71.
27. Wiggins JE, Patel SR, Shedden KA, et al. NFkappaB promotes inflammation, coagulation, and fibrosis in the aging glomerulus. J Am Soc Nephrol 2010; 21(4):587–97.
28. Smith-Vikos T, Slack FJ. MicroRNAs and their roles in aging. J Cell Sci 2012;125: 7–17.
29. Leung AK, Sharp PA. MicroRNA functions in stress responses. Mol Cell 2010;40: 205–15.
30. Karolina DS, Wintour EM, Bertram J, et al. Riboregulators in kidney development and function. Biochimie 2010;92(3):217–25.
31. Harvey SJ, Jarad G, Cunningham J, et al. Podocyte-specific deletion of Dicer alters cytoskeletal dynamics and causes glomerular disease. J Am Soc Nephrol 2008;19:2069–75.
32. Grillari J, Grillari-Voglauer R. Novel modulators of senescence, aging and longevity: small non-coding RNAs enter the stage. Exp Gerontol 2010;45(4):302–11.
33. Geanacopoulos M. The determinants in lifespan in the nematode Caenorhabditis elegans: a short primer. Sci Prog 2004;87(Pt 4):227–47.
34. Edgar D, Trifunovic A. The mtDNA mutator mouse: dissecting mitochondrial involvement in aging. Aging (Albany NY) 2009;1(12):1028–32.
35. Cuervo AM, Bergamini E, Brunk UT, et al. Autophagy and aging: the importance of maintaining "clean" cells. Autophagy 2005;1(3):131–40.
36. Hartleben B, Gödel M, Meyer-Schwesinger C, et al. Autophagy influences glomerular disease susceptibility and maintains podocyte homeostasis in aging mice. J Clin Invest 2010;120(4):1084–96.
37. Muller FL, Lustgarten MS, Jang Y, et al. Trends in oxidative aging theories. Free Radic Biol Med 2007;43(4):477–503.
38. Ferrucci L. The Baltimore Longitudinal Study of Aging (BLSA): a 50-year-long journey and plans for the future. J Gerontol A Biol Sci Med Sci 2008;63(12): 1416–9.
39. Vlassara H, Uribarri J, Ferrucci L, et al. Identifying advanced glycation end products as a major source of oxidants in aging: implications for the management and/or prevention of reduced renal function in elderly persons. Semin Nephrol 2009;29(6):594–603.

40. Makita Z, Yanagisawa K, Kuwajima S, et al. Advanced glycation endproducts and diabetic nephropathy. J Diabet Complications 1995;9(4):265–8.
41. Uribarri J, Peppa M, Cai W, et al. Restriction of dietary glycotoxins reduces excessive advanced glycation endproducts in renal failure patients. J Am Soc Nephrol 2003;14(3):728–31.
42. Navarro-Díaz M, Serra A, López D, et al. Obesity, inflammation, and kidney disease. Kidney Int Suppl 2008;(111):S15–8.
43. Muntner P, Coresh J, Smith JC, et al. Plasma lipids and risk of developing renal dysfunction: the atherosclerosis risk in communities study. Kidney Int 2000; 58(1):293–301.
44. Okamura DM, Pennathur S, Pasichnyk K, et al. CD36 regulates oxidative stress and inflammation in hypercholesterolemic CKD. J Am Soc Nephrol 2009;20(3): 495–505.
45. Wiggins JE, Goyal M, Wharram BL, et al. Antioxidant ceruloplasmin is expressed by glomerular parietal epithelial cells and secreted into urine in association with glomerular aging and high-calorie diet. J Am Soc Nephrol 2006;17(5): 1382–7.
46. Thornalley PJ. Advanced glycation end products in renal failure [review]. J Ren Nutr 2006;16(3):178–84.
47. Thornalley PJ. Use of aminoguanidine (Pimagedine) to prevent the formation of advanced glycation endproducts [review]. Arch Biochem Biophys 2003;419(1): 31–40.
48. Bolton WK, Cattran DC, Williams ME, et al, ACTION I Investigator Group. Randomized trial of an inhibitor of formation of advanced glycation end products in diabetic nephropathy. Am J Nephrol 2004;24(1):32–40.
49. Forbes JM, Yee LT, Thallas V, et al. Advanced glycation end product interventions reduce diabetes-accelerated atherosclerosis. Diabetes 2004;53(7): 1813–23.
50. Bakris GL, Bank AJ, Kass DA, et al. Advanced glycation end-product cross-link breakers. A novel approach to cardiovascular pathologies related to the aging process. Am J Hypertens 2004;17(12 Pt 2):23S–30S.
51. Sabbagh MN, Agro A, Bell J, et al. PF-04494700, an oral inhibitor of receptor for advanced glycation end products (RAGE), in Alzheimer disease. Alzheimer Dis Assoc Disord 2011;25(3):206–12.
52. Peng X, Ma J, Chen F, et al. Naturally occurring inhibitors against the formation of advanced glycation end-products. Food Funct 2011;2(6):289–301.
53. McCay CM, Crowell MF, Maynard LA. The effect of retarded growth upon the length of life span and upon the ultimate body size. Nutrition 1935;5:155.
54. Yu BP, Masoro EJ, McMahan CA. Nutritional influences on aging of Fischer 344 rats: 1. Physical, metabolic and longevity characteristics. J Gerontol 1985;40(6): 657–70.
55. Maeda H, Gleiser CA, Masoro EJ, et al. Nutritional influences on aging of Fischer 344 rats: II Pathology. J Gerontol 1985;40(6):671–88.
56. Masoro EJ. Dietary restriction and aging. J Am Geriatr Soc 1993;41:994–9.
57. Nadon NL. Of mice and monkeys: National Institute on Aging resources supporting the use of animal models in biogerontology research. J Gerontol A Biol Sci Med Sci 2006;61(8):813–5.
58. Colman RJ, Anderson RM, Johnson SC, et al. Caloric restriction delays disease onset and mortality in rhesus monkeys. Science 2009;325(5937):201–4.
59. Wiggins JE, Goyal M, Sanden SK, et al. Podocyte hypertrophy, "adaptation," and "decompensation" associated with glomerular enlargement and

glomerulosclerosis in the aging rat: prevention by calorie restriction. J Am Soc Nephrol 2005;16(10):2953–66.

60. Redman LM, Ravussin E. Caloric restriction in humans: impact on physiological, psychological, and behavioral outcomes. Antioxid Redox Signal 2011;14(2): 275–87.

Index

Note: Page numbers of article titles are in **boldface** type.

Clin Geriatr Med 29 (2013) 731–736
http://dx.doi.org/10.1016/S0749-0690(13)00052-9
0749-0690/13/$ – see front matter © 2013 Elsevier Inc. All rights reserved.

geriatric.theclinics.com

Printed and bound by CPI Group (UK) Ltd, Croydon, CR0 4YY

03/10/2024

01040408-0015